D1799814

Disclaimer

The information in this book is meant for educational purposes only in relation to the specific subjects addressed. It is not intended as, and should not be relied upon, as medical advice. It is not intended to replace or countermand the advice given by the reader's personal physician. The author and the publisher are not responsible for any adverse effects or consequences resulting from the use of the information in this book. It is the responsibility of the reader to consult a physician regarding his or her own personal care.

Date of publication: August 2019

Last review: August 2019

Cover photograph: Oliver Perrott

Contents

Foreward

Our health impacts us on a daily basis. Poor health can lead us to being unable to do the things we enjoy, spend time with the people we love or feel fulfilled with our lives.

In 2008 my world collapsed when I was diagnosed with the chronic long-term health condition ulcerative colitis. I thought my life was over and I was condemned to forever feeling a former shadow of myself. I was placed on strong medication and told I may face surgery to remove my colon in the future.

Fast forward 10 years and I'm now living a healthier life than I ever could have imagined for myself - even before my ulcerative colitis diagnosis. I am medication free, have never had surgery and am in clinical remission - things I never would have believed could have happened.

I often get asked by people how I've managed to do this. This book is my story of how I've taken control of my health and what I now do to stay well.

It's not intended to be a guide for other people to follow, I'm not a medical practitioner and we are all different in how we respond, but I hope it does inspire you to know that having a chronic condition doesn't mean you can't enjoy times of good health too.

Seb Tucknott

My story

On March 22, 2008 my life changed forever. That day was the first time I noticed blood. I was 21 and working away and when I went to the toilet there it was - blood on the toilet paper when I wiped. At the time I didn't think anything of it. I didn't realise that from then on my life was going to dramatically change. I just chucked the paper into the toilet bowl, flushed and carried on with my day.

Now I know that blood is your body's way of warning you that something is wrong, but, at the time I did what many people often do - ignored it and hoped it would go away.

Of course, it didn't. The blood continued for several days after I returned home to Brighton, and then I started experiencing bloody diarrhoea too. It was the urgency of needing to go to the toilet that actually made me think I should seek medical help, rather than the blood. I went to my GP and was told I had haemorrhoids, was given some cream (without an examination being done) and was sent on my way. I felt the diagnosis was wrong so I didn't use the cream and carried on for the next few days hoping the diarrhoea would stop on its own. But it didn't, it got worse. A lot worse.

So, back to the doctor I went and this time I was taken more seriously. I was given steroid enemas, a referral to a gastroenterologist for six weeks' time and a blood test.

By now I had started Googling and I was pretty sure I had ulcerative colitis. As the days passed while I waited for the appointment my symptoms got worse and worse. I struggled through the next few days, including playing the last game of the season for my football team.

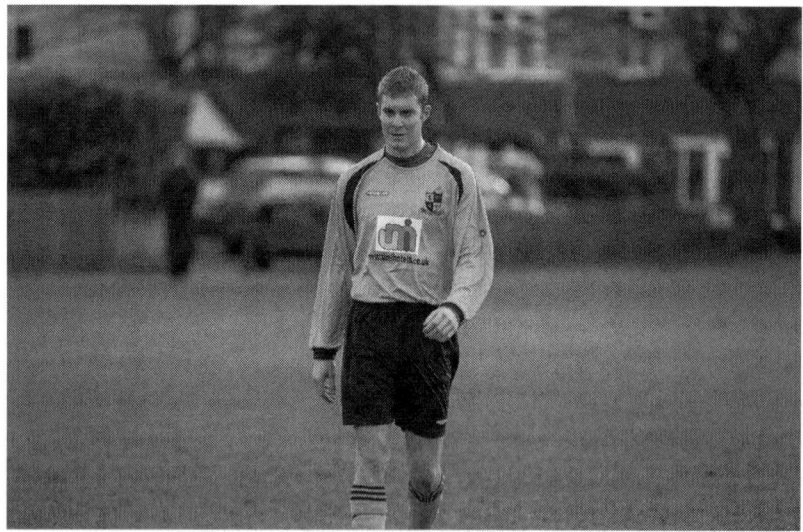

Playing football just before IBD diagnosis

But my symptoms continued to go downhill and I ended up going to Accident & Emergency. The doctor asked if I had a fever, I said no, and he said it can't be ulcerative colitis because it always presents with a fever. He also concluded I had haemorrhoids (again no examination) and sent me home.

A few days later I was still really struggling. I was going to the toilet every half hour. I wasn't eating or drinking because everything was just going through me and I had lost 10kgs in two weeks. My face was gaunt and my skin was grey. I hated looking at myself in the mirror. I couldn't cope and went back to A&E. I was living with my parents at the time and by this stage they were really worried. In the car on the way there we agreed that this time we wouldn't leave hospital until someone had properly examined me. But, we didn't need to be insistent. One of the first things the doctor who saw me did was carry out a digital examination. He didn't find any haemorrhoids but did find mucous. I was so relieved that someone had finally found something. I was sent to an assessment ward. My blood was taken (using a cannula and a syringe because I was so dehydrated), given a glucose drip and I spent the night there. But I couldn't sleep and I just walked up and down dragging my drip around. In the morning I was given an enema ready for a sigmoidoscopy.

"So many emotions came flooding out – relief they had found what was wrong with me and that I was going to be looked after, but also fear about the future"

The moment the video from the sigmoidoscopy came up on the screen I knew I had ulcerative colitis (UC). I could see the inflammation and it looked just like the pictures I had seen on Google. My colon was in a bad way and I was told I may need to have emergency surgery. They took biopsies and I was taken to the recovery ward. A nurse came over to talk to me, but I just burst into tears. So many emotions came flooding out – relief they had found what was wrong with me and that I was going to be looked after, but also fear about the future. I'd read so many negative things about UC online and I was scared. I didn't think I would be able to enjoy any of the things I had before again. Of course, I now know that's not the case, but no-one told me that at the time.

There was no room for me on the gastroenterology ward so I spent an interesting 24 hours on the amputee ward instead! I was given IV steroids (which work to reduce inflammation and suppress the immune system), an X-ray to check for blockages and afterwards was taken off nil-by-mouth. Thankfully the IV steroids started working pretty quickly and I didn't need to have any surgery.

In total I spent nine days in hospital. I was sent home with Pentasa (mesalazine - a medication which works to reduce inflammation in the gut) and oral corticosteroids (Prednisolone) and an appointment to see a gastroenterologist. The gastroenterologist talked briefly to me about what life with colitis would be like. The main thing that stuck in my mind was that he thought I probably wouldn't be able to exercise as much. Being active has always been a big part of my life. I love playing football, biking, skiing, snowboarding - so this was a big blow to think I may have to slow down. I was also told there would be a cure for UC within 5-20 years. I was referred for a colonoscopy and the result was severe pancolitis. No wonder I had been bleeding so badly, they said.

After being back at home for a while the diarrhoea and bleeding started to settle down. It was such a strange feeling being back at home. Even though I'd been away for less than two weeks it felt like a lifetime. Everyone was carrying on with their lives as normal. But for me my whole world had changed. I suddenly felt very different from everyone else. I gradually started to put weight back on and when I looked in the mirror I recognised myself again.

Returning to normal life - April 2008

Within days of returning home from hospital I was feeling so much better that I went to the park with my brother to play football, but I struggled to run. I was so unfit and fatigued that I could hardly move. Feeling this way was a huge shock and the doctor's words telling me I wouldn't be able to exercise as much rung in my ears.

I went back to work for the web design company my brother and I had set up. Money was tight and we didn't have many clients, so I wasn't really seeing anyone outside of my immediate family. Looking back now I think not having the opportunity to talk to people in the early days after my diagnosis didn't help me with the acceptance process. Perhaps if I had talked about it to someone, anyone, it would have helped the fact I had a chronic illness to sink in.

However, with the steroids doing such a good job, I was able to get back to doing most of the things I had been doing before. At times I almost forgot about my UC and I looked pretty 'normal' so the outside world didn't really know how sick I'd been (and how sick I could become again).

I knew that taking steroids long-term wasn't a great idea

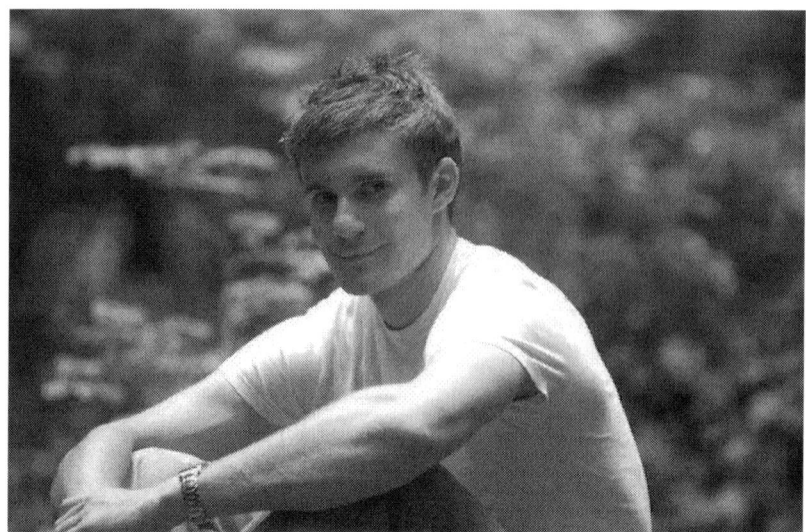

Just after diagnosis

because of the side effects they could have on me (such as osteoporosis and muscle weakness), but because I'd been told there would be a cure I think I became complacent. I just pinned all my hopes on a cure and decided I'd worry about the consequences of what I was doing to my body later down the line.

Now that my symptoms were under control I tried to taper down my steroids, as directed by the doctor. I was taking eight tablets (40mg) a day but every time I went below 20mg my symptoms would get worse. I'd start needing the toilet more, would see blood in the toilet bowl and I would have to increase the dose back up to 40mg to get it under control again. This vicious cycle continued for the first year.

In July 2008, just three months after my diagnosis, I met Emily.

At first I didn't really talk to her about my UC. On our first date we went for a walk and I mentioned I'd recently been in hospital and been diagnosed with IBD, but she'd never heard of it. She asked a few questions and then the subject would change. I think I gave her the impression that the medication was keeping it under control (which it was until I started to try to decrease it), that it wasn't that serious and everything would be OK because there would be a cure soon.

We did everything that 'normal' new couples would do. We went out for creamy Italian dinners, cocktails in trendy bars, shared a bottle of wine in front of a film. Knowing what I know now about my body I realise that none of this was any good for my colitis.

"I'd soiled myself and could feel it running down my leg, but I just kept quiet and carried on walking and talking"

It was on one of our first dates that I experienced my first public 'toilet accident'. I'd had a small accident while I was in hospital after having the sigmoidoscopy, but I blamed it on the air escaping that they had pumped into my body for the examination, along with some stool. Emily and I lived about a 10 minute walk from each other. We'd been for a walk along the beach and as we started to head back to her flat I felt the familiar, formidable feeling in my bowels. I tried to ignore it and carried on walking, but, when we were around 500m from Emily's flat, I didn't think I could hold on anymore. I had a short moment of internal panic before it was too late to take action. I'd soiled myself and could feel it running down my leg, but I just kept quiet and carried on walking and talking. When Emily reached her flat, I declined coming inside and carried on walking the 10 minutes to my own flat. It felt like miles. Relieved, I finally reached my building and got into the lift to go to my flat on the 3rd floor. At that point I caught a glimpse of myself in the mirror and saw that it had soaked through my trousers and was clearly visible for everyone to see. I was sure Emily would have realised what had happened and I was devastated. However, she didn't ever mention it, and it was only when we were talking seven years later that I told her what had happened and found out she was completely oblivious.

In the coming months there were a few more occasions where I had accidents between mine and Emily's homes. As a result I started making lots of negative associations with that walk, almost like a self-fulfilling prophecy, and each time I did it I believed I'd have an accident...so I did (well not every time, but it certainly felt that way!).

My car would also become a regular toilet for me. I'm lucky that because I have my own company I can choose where my office is and have made it a short walk from my home. This means I don't have to endure a long commute. However, I often used to have to travel for 20 minutes or more by car to visit clients. It would always be on these car journeys, when I knew I had no access to a toilet, that I would need it most. I would often sit on a plastic bag and carry a boot full of spare clothes in anticipation that I'd need the toilet and not be able to stop somewhere suitable in time.

Thankfully my UC is under better control at the moment and it's not often that I have to rush to the toilet - let alone have an accident.

In January 2009 I was still struggling to cut down on the steroids. At this point my steroid 'moon face' was well established, as was an outrageous appetite. Some days I'd have a full fry up for breakfast and then just half an hour later several bowls of cereal. I'd also work my way through bags of sweets, cakes, biscuits, packaged sandwiches, pasta and pizza. If I ate any fruit, vegetables or salads I'd find myself on the toilet only minutes later. At the time I didn't really think about what this diet was doing to my insides (the fact that our bodies need fibre and nutrients to function didn't even cross my mind). I was just happy to be eating. I was only focusing on trying to get as many calories as possible.

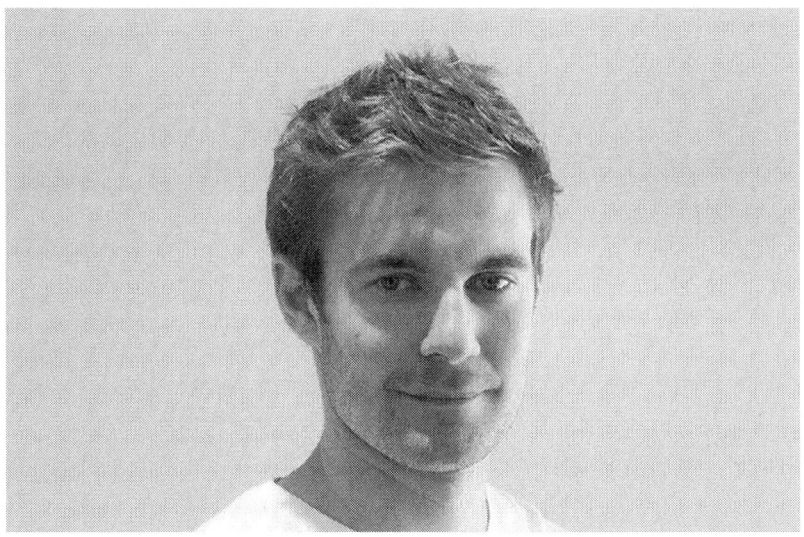

My moon face and very unhealthy skin

With my UC still out of control and unable to come off the steroids I also started taking the immunosuppressant Azathioprine (which works to suppress the immune system) too. Around this time I also went on my first holiday with Emily (and her friends), a snowboarding trip to Les Deux Alpes in France. I felt awful the whole time but I didn't want to ruin Emily's trip so I didn't say anything. I was determined to snowboard and not let my UC get in the way. And I did join in. I also started playing football again, but taking the Azathioprine just didn't make me feel like myself. I was paranoid about getting colds and I felt constantly run down and tired. I continued to take it for around six months but my consultant and I decided to stop it because it wasn't working well enough for me to taper off the steroids.

So, I carried on with the steroids and settled into a seemingly endless cycle of trying to drop the dose, which would cause my symptoms to get worse, so would need to up the dose again. Then, towards the end of the year, I suddenly managed to stop taking steroids completely, and for around nine months was just on Pentasa. There didn't seem to be a reason why I'd suddenly managed it but it felt great to finally lose the moon face and drop some weight. But, in June 2010 I got an abscess in my tooth which I had to take antibiotics for. This triggered one of my worst flares to begin and out came the steroids again.

For all the time that I've had colitis I have run my own company. This has been both a blessing and a curse. It's a blessing because it has given me the flexibility to stay at home on the toilet or have an afternoon nap when I've been unwell, and a curse because it causes me a lot of stress.

Some of the worst flares I've had have been triggered by a stressful event, and all these stressful events have been work-related. I flared badly after my business partner left the company, when I had to make several people redundant, when I haven't been able to pay staff and when there was too much work to do (or too little). The stress has never gone away, but I've never wanted to give up my company so I've had to learn a lot of coping strategies to help me deal with it. I now have a pretty full armoury of coping mechanisms which I have to regularly delve into to keep my equilibrium (I'll explain more about this, which I call my 'balance theory', later).

"I was concerned my UC wouldn't behave and I would be ill on my wedding day or I would delay the ceremony because I was on the toilet"

In May 2010 Emily proposed to me and we set our wedding day for March 1, 2011. Neither of us wanted a big, glitzy wedding so we decided to get married in the ski resort Meribel in the French Alps with just a few family and friends. We chose a clearing which had an amazing view looking out over the valley (and which was near to some toilets!). In the run up to the big day I started to get anxiety. I was concerned my UC wouldn't behave and I would be ill on my wedding day or I would delay the ceremony because I was on the toilet. It's probably the worst fear of many people I speak with who have IBD and are getting married.

We arrived in Meribel on February 27th and were set to be

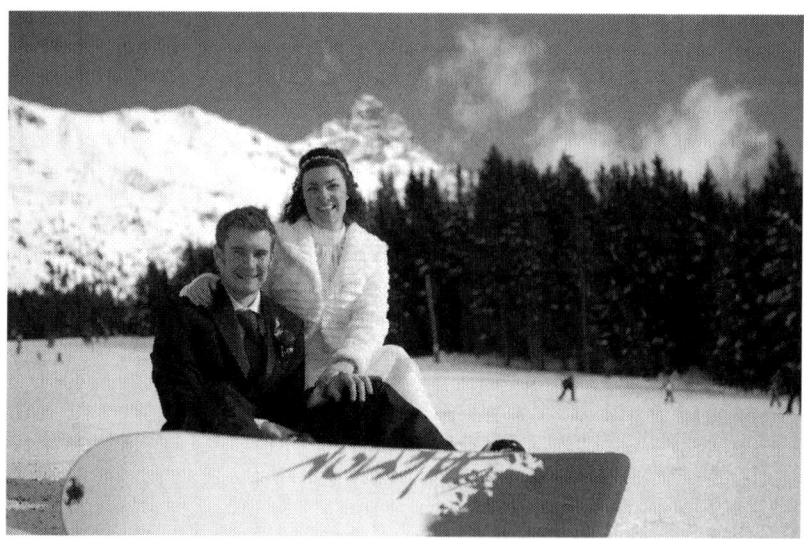

Our wedding

married two days later. We were staying in a beautiful cha-
let with all our nearest and dearest under the one roof. Sure
enough, the night before the wedding my stomach started
playing up and by the early hours of the morning I was on
and off the toilet every half an hour. By the morning I was
just passing water and I was feeling very weak. At around
5am I had to tell Emily that I couldn't go through with the
wedding. I was devastated but I was too ill. A little later she
went downstairs to tell everyone, only to come back up-
stairs not long after to say that everyone was ill in bed with
a sickness bug. I felt so relieved! It wasn't my UC playing
up, I'd just caught the sickness bug too. Luckily we were
able to move the wedding to a few days later on March 4th
and by then most people were feeling better (albeit a little
thinner and weaker from several days of diarrhoea and
vomiting!).

I did almost miss Emily's arrival at our wedding though because, on-route, I had to make an emergency dash to the toilet in a mountain-side bar. My best man was worried, but after the events of the past few days I wasn't fazed. I survived the rest of the day without any more urgent toilet trips. Every time I look at the photos from our wedding day I'm reminded of the huge amount of steroids I was taking at the time. My 'moon face' is evident for everyone to see. I hate seeing it but also enjoy realising how far I've now come from that time.

Life changing moments - 2012

So, by now I knew that stress was a huge trigger for making my symptoms worse, and I had discovered some other things too. I avoided eating tomatoes, salad leaves, grapes and anything else with tough skins and seeds as I would see all of these go straight through me and end up in the toilet. I also knew that alcohol wasn't good for me (though I still drank it a little). I had accepted this was how it was going to be - well, until they found that cure I was promised! In the summer of 2012, still struggling to keep my flares under control, my consultant added 6-Mercaptopurine (another immunosuppressant which works to suppress the immune system) to the medications I was taking as he wanted me off of steroids. I agreed to take it, but was pretty nervous having read articles online about some of the side effects. I was also aware that it was in the same category of drugs as azathioprine - and that hadn't previously worked for me. As a result I never felt comfortable taking it, and spent the whole time just really wanting to come off it.

Then a cliche, life-changing moment happened during the London 2012 Olympics. I've always enjoyed athletics and I competed when I was younger until I got Osgood-Schlatter disease in my knees, which made it painful to train. Watching the Games reminded me of how much I missed athletics. So I decided, there and then, that I was going to start training again. I joined Brighton Athletics Club and found I was still pretty good. My times weren't bad and there was lots of room for improvement.

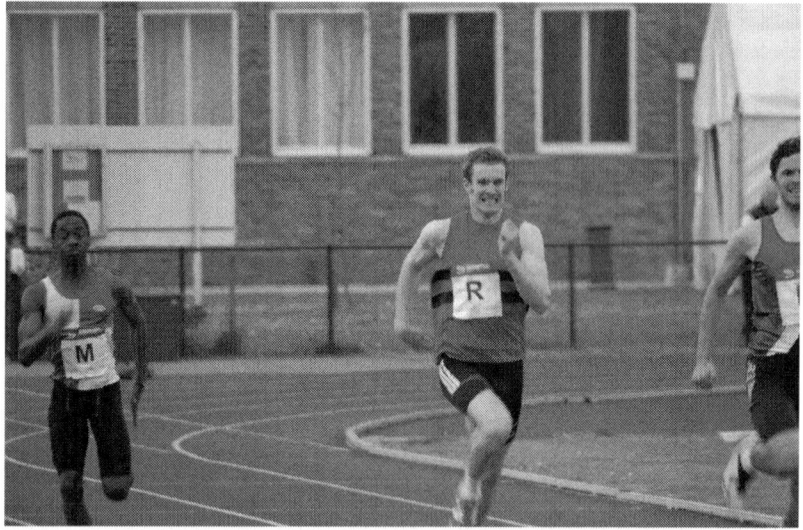

Running for Brighton & Hove

At the same time I also found my colitis symptoms started to improve, and not just the toilet-related ones. My muscles and joints were aching less and I had more energy. My mother is Finnish and as my times steadily improved I decided I wanted to try to run for Finland. However, to compete at a national level I thought I would need to come off my steroid medication.

Around the same time, at a family social event, I got talking to a friend of my brother's who is an acupuncturist about my steroid dilemma. He said he could help and in November 2012 I went to see him as a patient. I have a science background (I studied chemical engineering at university) and have never really been a believer in alternative medicine, but my desire to get off the steroids was so great that I was willing to give anything a go. The treatment was incredibly relaxing (there were several times I fell asleep) and I always felt great after leaving. He told me I had too much 'heat' and 'damp' in my body and the acupuncture was trying to reduce that. He told me to stop eating gluten, dairy, sugar, caffeine and nightshades (potatoes, tomatoes, aubergines, peppers) if I wanted to really help myself. He said all of those foods caused 'damp' and 'heat'. Again, I decided I had nothing to lose by trying it. Emily was already being very supportive in adapting the foods we ate to suit my colitis but when I told her I was no longer eating gluten, dairy or nightshades I remember her asking what we could actually eat. However, once she got used to the idea, she embraced it fully. I continued with the acupuncture treatments for a while and the diet seemed to be having an effect. I was able to start weaning myself off the steroids.

Then, in January 2013 I was able to come off the 6-Mercaptopurine and the steroids at the same time (and I haven't been back on them since). In May I became Sussex Champion in 200m and 400m and in July I went on a mountain biking holiday to the French Alps.

Sadly, I haven't reached my goal of competing for Finland. Work and having a baby in 2015 have distracted me, but I'm still training and enjoying it (and it's still having huge benefits for stress-relief and helping my joint and muscle pains too).

"I still have some bad days but the good days greatly outweigh them"

Since then I've done a lot of research into why giving up gluten and dairy has worked for me (more on this later in the book). I am eating nightshades again without problem but I do now also limit the amount of grains, sugar and processed food I eat. I don't drink much alcohol (if I do it will generally be red wine or gluten free beer) and try to only drink filtered water. I've also been able to reintroduce all fruit, vegetables, nuts and seeds into my diet, including being able to eat them raw. Although I didn't continue the acupuncture treatments for long (I couldn't afford them and I wasn't sure how much effect they were having) there have been a hundred or so other small changes I've made in my life. These have included practising mindfulness, having an air filter at home, improving my sleep and using a standing desk at work, which I believe collectively have had a positive effect on my health, and in turn on my colitis.

I still have some bad days but the good days greatly outweigh them. Over the years I've learnt to manage my flares better and am incredibly strict with looking after myself when I feel like I'm heading towards a flare. It's also led me to create my 'balance theory', which you can read about in 'My balance theory' section of this book.

Was I in remission? - 2016

In 2016 my wife and I launched the IBDrelief website (www.ibdrelief.com). During my research into IBD I'd found there was very little information or support available for people who wanted to learn more about their condition and ways to support self-management of their IBD. What I'd learnt about IBD and my own health had helped me so much that I wanted a place to share the information and for people to share their own thoughts on how they manage their condition.

Feeling better also allowed me the energy to work on IBDrelief alongside my day job. But, despite my symptoms being stable for a couple of years I didn't have any confirmation that things were going OK on the inside of my body. So, when I was called to hospital in January 2016 for a colonoscopy (a camera which views your colon) I was pretty nervous. What if all the changes I'd done, all the hard work I'd put in had been for nothing? And, for the first few moments of the colonoscopy I thought that was the case. There was obvious inflammation in the rectum and transverse colon, but as the endoscope moved further up my colon and reached the transverse bend there was nothing, no ulcers, no inflammation, nothing. I came away with a diagnosis of mild to moderate proctosigmoiditis. To say I was elated is an understatement, and seeing how happy my family were made me even more determined to keep up my new lifestyle.

"To say I was elated is an understatement, and seeing how happy my family were made me even more determined to keep up my new lifestyle"

As the months passed I carried on making lots of small changes to keep my health in the best place possible. I started to feel better and better and would forget about my colitis for weeks, so much so that I was forgetting to take my Pentasa. Eventually I stopped taking this too. I felt great for around 6 months but then I had a flare. I was incredibly stressed at work and wasn't sleeping. My diet had also slipped, I got a cold and my immune system was low. I was due to cycle the South Down's Way (100 mile off-road cycle) for charity in 10 days' time and I was worried I wouldn't be able to make it through. However, I focused on my health by going to bed early, eating nutritiously and de-stressing and I made it through the flare and through the bike ride.

During that period I had a calprotectin test done, with a result of over 300. Calprotectin is a substance your body releases into your poo when inflammation is present. Generally results under 50 are considered clear (as most of us produce some levels of calprotectin) and between 50-200 are borderline, so my result showed that I definitely had some inflammation present. Six months later I had another and it was back down to 60. To make sure things were still OK my consultant was keen for me to have another colonoscopy. So in November 2017 I was back in the endoscopy unit, and again I was nervous. Having only recently been through a bad flare with a high calprotectin level I was sure that things wouldn't look good, even though I was back to feeling great again. However, I couldn't have been more wrong. Things looked even better than they had nearly two years previously. There was no sign of inflammation at all and I was told I was in clinical remission.

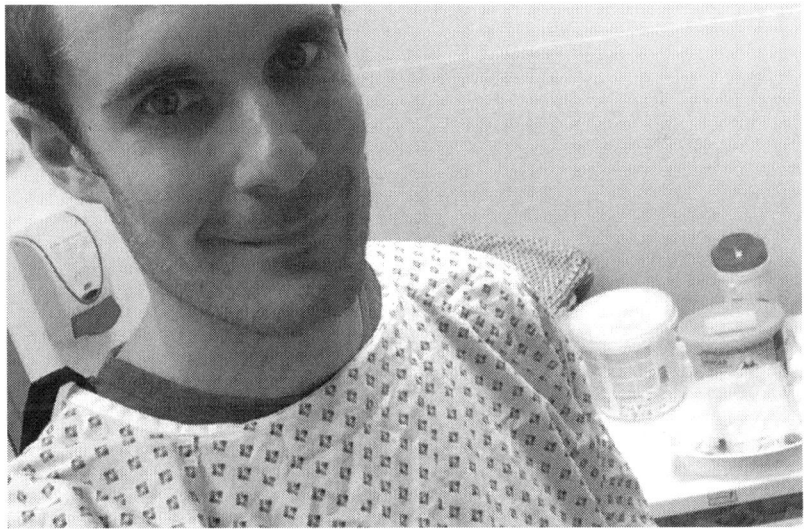

Ready for my endoscopy

Since then I haven't had another significant flare and I can honestly say I have never felt as good as I feel now (even before my colitis) but life can be unpredictable and I know this doesn't mean that things won't change in the future. Right now though, I'm just enjoying every day while I can. I believe that by supporting my body to be in the best health it can possibly be I've helped my colitis to reach remission and am giving myself every opportunity to stay that way for as long as possible.

"Things looked even better than they had nearly two years previously. There was no sign of in-flammation at all and I was told I was in clinical remission"

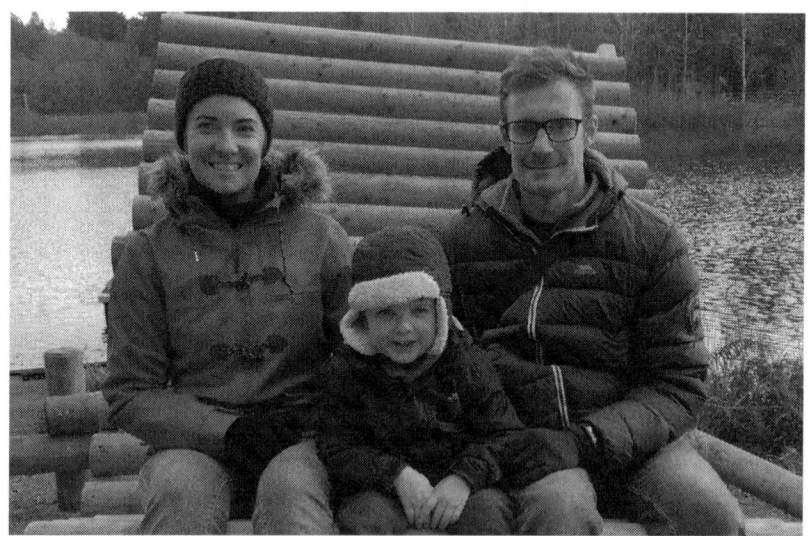

My little family

My balance theory

I started practising my 'balance theory' subconsciously before I actually realised what I was doing. It's something I have organically developed over time and which has been truly life-changing for me. I hope my descriptions of it in this chapter do it the justice it deserves.

In 2012, after visiting an acupuncturist, making some changes to my diet and starting athletics training (read more about all this in my story in 'My story'), I began doing a lot of reading about IBD and UC. I started out by reading all the general stuff available on medical and charity sites (such as the NHS and Crohn's & Colitis UK) and when I ran out of this information I began delving into medical literature and research. It sounds strange but, despite being diagnosed 4 years previously, I hadn't really paid that much attention to what IBD was other than the very basic facts.

At the same time as doing this reading I started to become more in tune with my body and notice that some things I was doing affected my health negatively and other things were having a positive affect. Obviously, once I realised this, I began trying to do as much of the good stuff as I could and as little of the bad.

As time passed I discovered more things to put into both the good and bad columns. Six years on I'm still discovering new things and it has become an ever-evolving process.

"I started to become more in tune with my body and notice that some things I was doing affected my health negatively and other things were having a positive affect"

It sounds so simple and straightforward but it has required a lot of effort and willpower to get to the stage I'm at now (and also learning to accept that some things are outside of my control).

Looking back on things it's great to see how my 'balance' has evolved as I've become more aware of the things that affect me. Here is an example of what it looked like just after I'd been diagnosed in 2008 (although at the time I was ignorant to the things that made me worse - which I now feel affected my ability to come off of steroids).

Things that made me better (good)	Things that made me worse (bad)
Prednisolone steroids	Stress
Pentasa	Certain foods
	Worry about my health

My 'balance' after diagnosis

Following advice from my consultant, the next step was to try another medication to support the "good" side and I was given Azathioprine to try. After reading about the side effects of Azathioprine and wondering what this drug may

do to me my stress and worry levels increased. I also started to feel run down and not myself.

This made my new 'balance' look like this:

Things that made me better (good)	Things that made me worse (bad)
Prednisolone steroid	More stress
Pentasa	Certain foods
Azathioprine	More worry about my health

My 'balance' after being prescribed Azathioprine

So, even though I had added something to my 'good' side, I
had made my 'bad' side bigger too. This again meant every
time I tried to come off the steroids my balance became unbalanced and my UC got worse. Back to square one!
I went through this cycle for four-and-a-half years, also
trying the medication 6-mercaptopurine, again with the
same results. I knew being on Prednisolone forever wasn't
an option and was already suffering the effects of long-term
use such as 'moon face', acne, signs of osteoporosis, mood
swings and excessive sweating. It was time to try a different
approach!

So, against my better judgement I went to see an acupuncturist. As well as the relaxing treatments he advised me
to rethink my diet and try excluding gluten, dairy, sugar,
nightshades, caffeine and alcohol from my diet. So, I went

cold turkey and started straight away. I also started doing athletics training. And, it all did make me feel better, to the point that I was able to taper off the steroids completely.

My new balance now looked like this:

Things that made me better (good)	Things that made me worse (bad)
Pentasa	Stress
New diet	Some worry
Athletics training	

My 'balance' after changing my diet and starting athletics training

I kept up the acupuncture for about 6 months. I wasn't convinced it was doing anything, although it was nice to have 45 minutes' relaxing time once a week. I am really glad I tried it though as it led me down the path I'm on now. More recently I've learnt more about how acupuncture works and I would try it again in the future if I felt I needed to.

Since then I've refined my diet and changed many aspects of my lifestyle that allow me to now feel healthier than I've ever felt and live symptom free 95% of the time.

Now, whenever my symptoms get worse instead of reaching for a packet of steroids straight away I quickly identify what in my balance has changed and either fix it or compensate for it. Every time I've recovered quicker and quicker. Over time I've developed more knowledge, strategies and confidence to help me when I feel my health is deteriorating. And, I have the added reassurance of knowing that the steroids, or other medications, will always be there to give me a little helping hand should things go too far.

It's worth mentioning at this point that many people believe that because I now live medication free I am against using medication to treat IBD. This is absolutely not the case. Medication saves lives. It stopped me from losing my colon and allowed me to get to the place I am today. It helps many people reach remission and stay there and have a better quality of life. If my health took a nosedive in the future then I would have no issues whatsoever with taking medication again, whether that be steroids or one of the newer biologic medications now available, to help bring me back to an equilibrium.

As I said earlier, my balance is ever-evolving and I know there's still plenty of other things to add in the future. Since starting out on this journey I've become more and more open to trying out new things and experimenting with how they make me feel. I now do things that 10 years ago I would have laughed at, such as meditation. Some people around me probably think I've become a bit obsessed with getting my health and wellbeing as optimal as possible. But, I don't think I am. Why would you not want to feel the best you possibly could? My energy levels are now through the roof, I'm incredibly happy and I wake up everyday looking forward to what lies ahead. If you would have told me five years ago that it was possible to feel this

"Medication saves lives. It stopped me from losing my colon and allowed me to get to the place I am today"

good then I wouldn't have believed you. But, even though I'm in remission, and feeling better than I ever have, I'm still constantly striving for even better health. I'm a perfectionist in everything I do, and my health is no different.

However, don't think I don't allow myself some treats (dark chocolate is my biggest downfall!) at times or that I don't slip up. It happens, I'm human. If I do overindulge though, my health soon reminds me and I return back to doing more of the good things in my balance than the bad.

So, how does the balance work in practice?

For me to be feeling well the stuff I'm doing from the good side of my balance has to be outweighing what's going on from the bad side. If it doesn't then my health starts deteriorating.

I mentioned earlier that if my symptoms start increasing (such increased toilet trips, increased gas, muscle pains, fatigue) I analyse my good and bad list and consider what things have changed recently. I then make adjustments to what I'm doing to try to get the good side above the bad side. Sometimes it may just be a case of improving one thing on my good list (such as getting some early nights because I've not been sleeping well) but often I have to work at several things to ensure the balance is tipped back in my favour. Everything also has a weighting. For example, from experience I know that sleep and stress are two of the biggest influences on my health. When I'm getting good sleep and have little stress my health is in a fairly good place and I can relax a bit with some of the other things on my 'good' list. However, as soon as one (or both) of these are affected things begin to go downhill. So, if I've had some restless nights or a stressful event I will be really strict with myself on things from my good list, such as the food I'm eating and making sure I'm relaxing and exercising.

"From experience I know that sleep and stress are two of the biggest influences on my health"

Sometimes I am able to predict when there will be a negative change in my health. This might be because I have a big project coming up at work that I need to get finished, or I've got a few evening events coming up which mean I'm not going to get as much sleep. By being aware of this I can start increasing the good things I am doing before the sleep deprivation and stress take an effect on my body. It's an art rather than a science and over the years I've learnt to become very in tune with my body and am constantly looking ahead to predict what things coming up in my diary may affect me.

I also constantly view my health like a bank balance. I'm aiming to build up a buffer in my account in case I hit hard times and need to dip into my savings. Every positive thing

I do for my health helps to add to this buffer and means that sometimes I can make withdrawals by doing some of the negative things (or not doing as many of the good things). But, as soon as I've spent this buffer I'll end up in my overdraft and my health starts to become affected. The longer I leave myself in my overdraft without doing positive things for my health the more in debt I get, and this is when my health seriously starts to suffer.

I have experimented with just trying to focus on one or two areas in my 'good' list and doing them as well as I possibly can, for example following my diet to the letter and meditating 3 times a day. But, although I was putting 100% effort into both of these areas I was not seeing improvements in my health, in fact I would sometimes see a deterioration. However, if I put 50% effort into the majority of the things on my 'good' side I saw a distinct improvement in my health that was longer lasting. So, for me, trying to do everything to some degree is better than doing a couple of things really well and ignoring the rest.

Differing states of health

I now have 3 potential states that my balance could be in:

1. Healthy/remission
2. Unstable/likely to flare
3. Declining health/flare up

Healthy/remission balance

When I'm doing more 'good' things than 'bad things' I'm in my healthy/remission state. The longer I can stay in this state the more stable my health becomes.

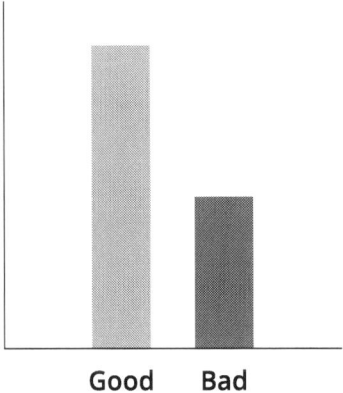

Good   Bad

Healthy/remission balance

Unstable/likely to flare balance

When I'm doing an equal amount of 'good' and 'bad' things I'm in my unstable/likely to flare state and one small change can tip the balance either way.

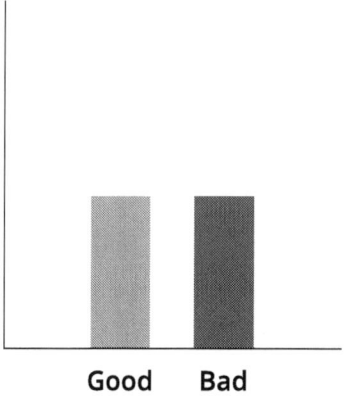

Good   Bad

Unstable/likely to flare balance

Declining health/flare up balance

When I'm doing more 'bad' things than 'good' things I'm in my declining health/flare up state. The longer I stay in this state the worse and longer a flare lasts.

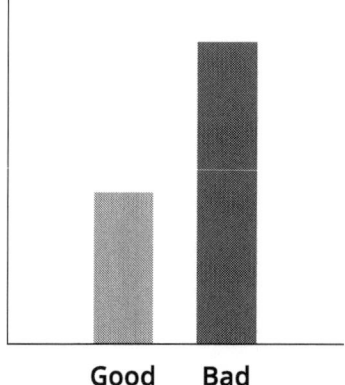

Good   Bad

Declining health/flare balance

Making health shifts

Significant change

If my bad side is greatly outweighing the good then just making one change to something on my good side is not enough to tip the balance back. I may need to combine several things to increase my good balance and ensure things from my bad side aren't holding me back. For example, I may work to improve my sleep routine but I might also be very stressed and not eating well so the improvements to my sleep are not making any difference. However, when I keep my improved sleep routine and work to decrease my stress levels the good column starts to outweigh the bad and my health starts to improve. In my early days of learning about my balance I would just do one thing (such as meditating) at a time and wouldn't see a difference so I'd stop doing it. Now I realise that it wasn't working because my bad column was outweighing the good column so much that it didn't tip the balance. It didn't mean that the thing I was doing wasn't having any positive effect, just not enough of an effect on its own to make a difference. If my health is declining I now keep layering up my 'good' things until my health starts tipping into the other direction.

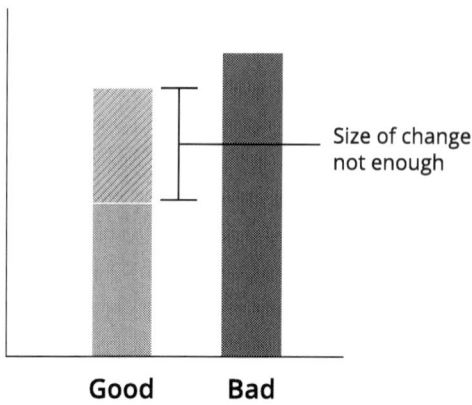

Good　　Bad

Change

Size of change not enough

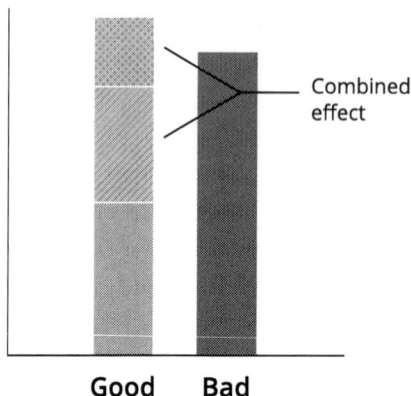

Good　　Bad

Change 1

Change 2

Combined effect of changes

Side effect

Some things may have both a positive effect and a negative effect. For example, when I started taking azathioprine any of the positive effects it may have been having were outweighed by the anxiety I had about the side effects of taking the medication. Another example is alcohol, which gives me enjoyment (therefore adds to my good side) but it's also a toxin that my body has to work hard to get rid of (therefore adds to my bad side).

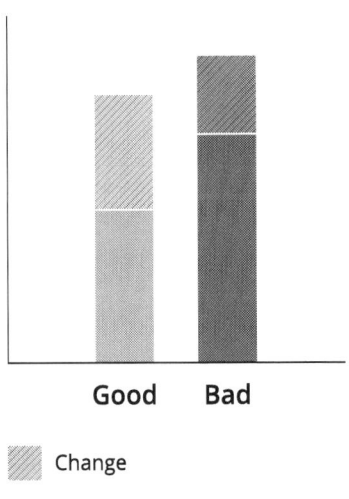

Good   **Bad**

Change

Side effect

Some 'good' things have a 'bad' side effect or vice versa

Dual effect

Some things I do have a dual effect, for example, exercising has a positive effect on my 'good' column but it also has the effect of reducing stress in my 'bad' column.

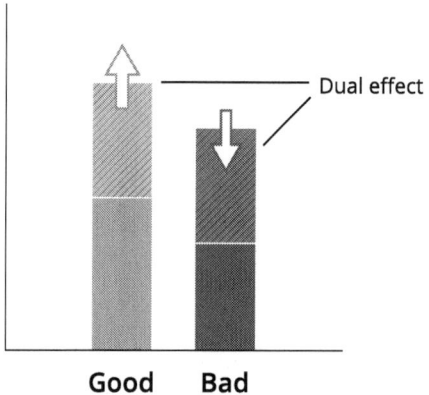

Good   **Bad**

Some things can have a positive dual effect (or a negative dual effect)

How a flare up can develop quickly

If I ignore my balance for a while then things can quickly escalate and before I know it I'm facing a flare up. It usually happens like this...

I am in a stable position (my good side is outweighing the bad) and something would then happen (e.g. a stressful event, super late night) so my bad side starts to outweigh my good side, even if it's just slightly.

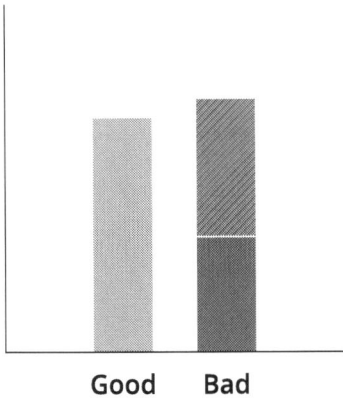

Good   Bad

 Change e.g. stressful situation

Balance suddenly changes so 'bad' outweighs 'good'

Now that my bad side is greater than the good side I may start to experience symptoms and my health starts to decline. This can then impact my good side because I may feel a bit more tired so I won't exercise as much, therefore making my balance even worse.

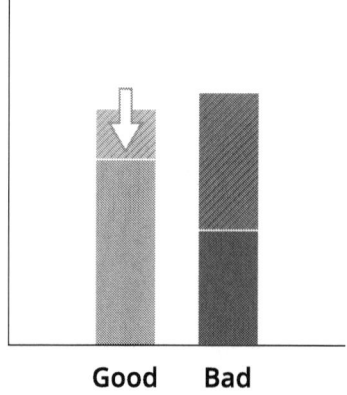

Good   Bad

 Change 2 e.g. less exercise

As I feel worse it affects my 'good' balance

Because I'm feeling worse I would then worry I'm having a flare up, my anxiety would increase, adding even more to my bad side. My health would be declining further so then my sleep would be affected because I'd be going to the toilet in the night, so my balance was getting even worse and then I'd find myself in a flare.

From this it's easy to see how you can go from a reasonable/good place to a bad place very quickly. Now that I've realised this I try to be proactive and increase my good things when I feel my health starting to decline.

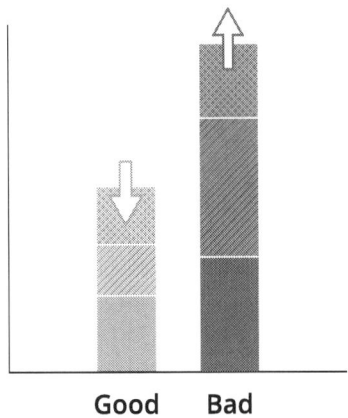

Good   **Bad**

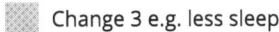 Change 3 e.g. less sleep

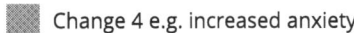 Change 4 e.g. increased anxiety

Changes can happen very quickly

Cumulative effect

As I mentioned earlier I tend to describe my health as being like a bank balance. Each day I pay some money in (by doing good things) and withdraw some money (by doing some 'bad' things). Over time if I've been paying in more money than withdrawing money I build up some savings, which I can then borrow at another time. However, if I borrow more than is in the account and go into my overdraft I reach the point of a flare.

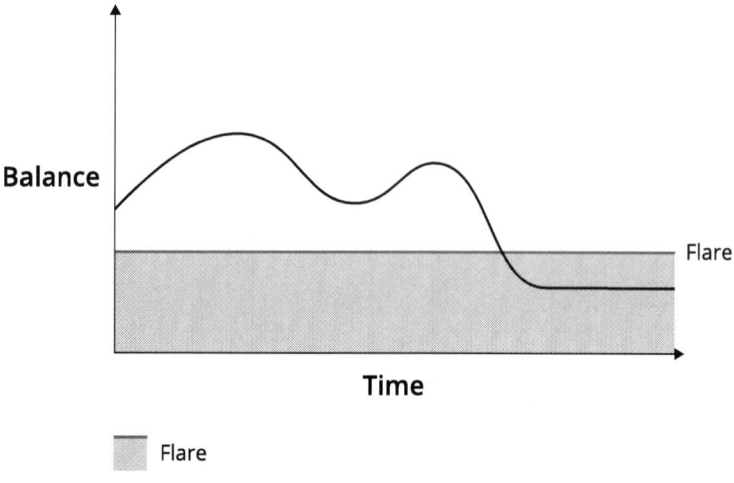

If I borrow more than I pay in my health dips below the flare line

Cumulative effect - Loan

For me I now see medication like a bank loan. When I go into my overdraft (a flare) I can use medication as if it were a loan to help push my health back quickly into a positive balance.

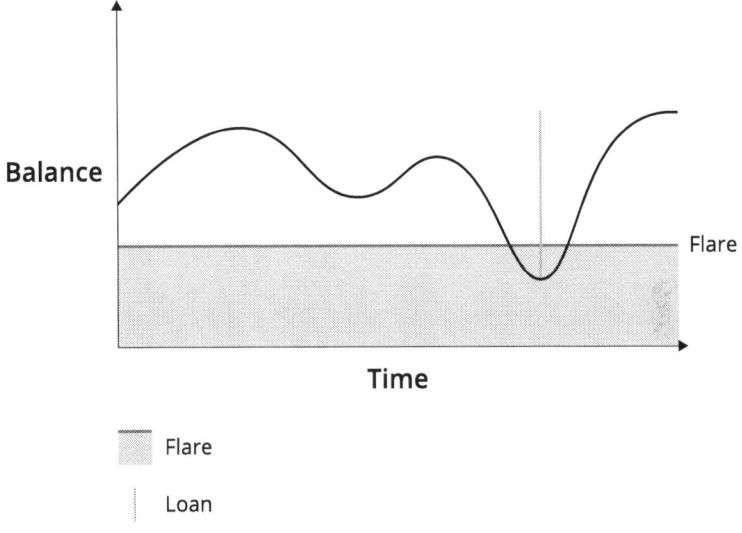

I view medication like a bank loan to pull me out of a flare and get me into remission

Reactive change

If I have a series of bad days I have now become in tune with my body and can quickly notice the symptoms of my health declining. At this point I will react to these symptoms by making a change, such as having a week of early nights.

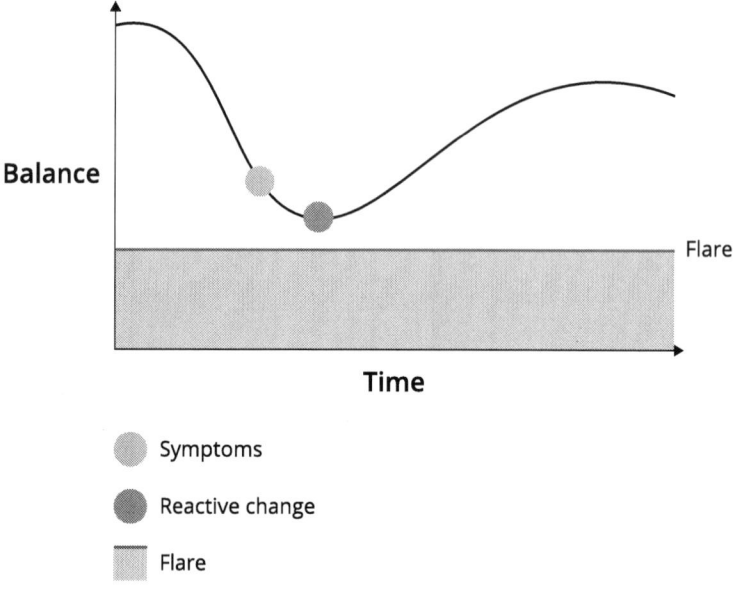

Balance

Flare

Time

- Symptoms
- Reactive change
- Flare

Making reactive changes can help my declining health to recover

Proactive change

Sometimes I'm aware of an event coming up with is likely to impact on my health, such as a big project at work which I'll need to work long hours. In this case I'll increase the number of things in my good column before the event to build up the reserve in my bank balance so that I have enough in there to cope with the event. Just like saving for a holiday, If I hadn't have done this my health would have more than likely declined so much that I would have a flare up.

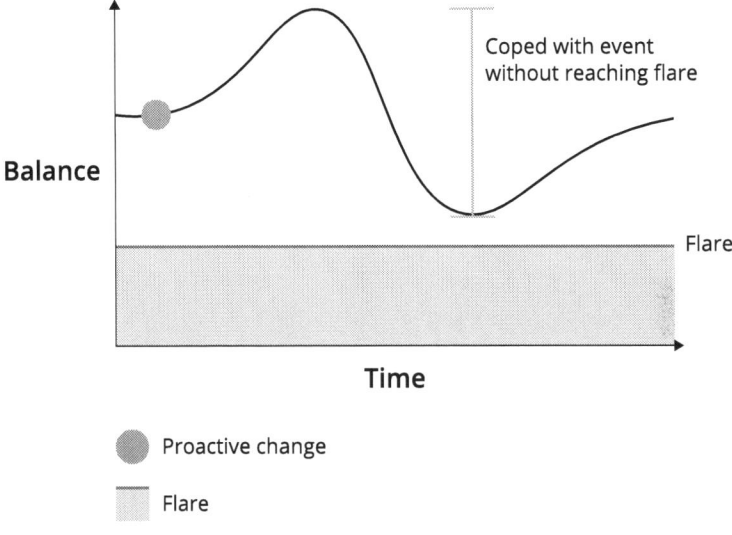

Making changes proactively helps me cope with events which will negatively effect me

The elements

But, I've learnt that it's not just as simple as having 'good' and 'bad' things. Each of these things can also be split into five different elements:

- Sleep
- Mind and stress
- Movement
- Diet
- Environment

To ensure my health remains stable I need to make sure that I'm doing things from each of these elements to keep things balanced. If I'm not doing enough of a range of things, and a couple of them drop below a certain point, then I will start to flare. Even if I'm doing everything I possibly can in one area this wouldn't be enough to keep me healthy. It's better to do a broad range of things across all the elements rather than excelling in just one area.

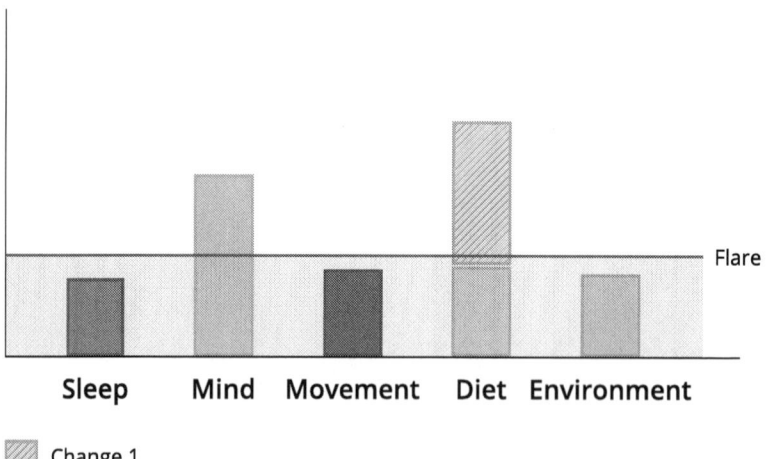

Flare

Sleep   Mind   Movement   Diet Environment

Change 1

Only focusing on one or two elements can mean I head towards a flare

So, here are some of the specific things I've discovered that are 'good' and 'bad' for my health broken down into the five elements...

Sleep

Things that positively affect my sleep (good)	Things that negatively affect my sleep (bad)
Evening technology detox	Disturbed sleep
Evening bath	Blue light in evenings (screens, bright lights)
Evening walk/run/cycle	Working late
Mindfulness & meditation	Noise during night
Magnesium supplements, spray and bath salts	Uncomfortable bed
Melatonin supplement	Illness
Saunas	Alcohol
	Pain
	Eating late
	Being too hot

Mind/Stress

Things that positively affect my mind/stress levels (good)	Things that negatively affect my mind/stress levels (bad)
Spending time with family/friends	General stress

Spending time with my son	Worrying about my UC
Holidays (and spa breaks)	Worrying about finding a toilet
Taking a proper lunch break	Worrying about money
Essential oils diffused around the house	Working too much
Mindfulness & meditation	
Walks	
Cycling	
Running	
Saunas	

Movement

Things that positively affect me physically (good)	Things that negatively affect me physically (bad)
Exercise	Sitting for long periods
Going for a walk	Lack of exercise
Yoga/pilates	Poor sleep
Massage	Pain
Using standing desk	

Barefoot shoes	
HIIT/Interval training	
Good sleep	

Diet

Things that positively affect my health (good)	Things that negatively affect my health (bad)
Vegetables	Gluten
Fruit	Tap water
Fish	Too much alcohol
Unprocessed meats	Dairy
Nuts	Processed foods
Seeds	Too many carbs
Herbs & spices	Sugar
Turmeric	Certain fats (vegetable oils, seed oils)
Filtered water	
Symprove probiotic	
Vitamin D supplement	

Magnesium supplement	
MSM supplement	
L-glutamine supplement	
Colostrum supplement	
Certain fats (coconut oil, olive oil)	

Environment

Things that positively affect my health (good)	Things that negatively affect my health (bad)
Filtered air	Taking antibiotics
Filtered water	Other illnesses (such as colds & coughs)
Natural deodorant	Exposure to chemicals (e.g. DIY/ cleaning)
Natural toothpaste	Pollution
Natural shampoo/conditioner/ soaps	Pollen
Organic food	

I'm at a place now that as long as I'm doing more of the good things than the bad then my health remains in a good place. Every one of these things has a different level of effect on me, for example, if I'm stressed this affects my health a lot more than if I have a glass or two of red wine. During times of stress I need to make sure I'm really focusing on doing as many of the good things as possible so my balance isn't upset.

This list is highly personal for me and if you applied it to yourself you would probably find that all these things would affect you differently. However, it's taken me years of experimenting to put together and I hope that by sharing it with you it may give you a head start to find your own lists want to give it a go. I've also found the order in which I do things is important. For example, I needed to make my room darker and quieter and get a more comfortable mattress before my sleep could improve. I can't promise this approach would work for anyone else though!

I'm aware that the majority of these things may not have a direct link to helping my IBD or have any evidence to show that they can help IBD. However, many of them do have some evidence to show they support general health. I feel it's incredibly important to make sure my body is in the best shape and the healthiest it possibly can be so all of its energy is focused on fighting my IBD instead of having other issues in my body that also need fixing. When explaining this to people I often refer to my body as a village. Imagine that there's been a murder in the village (my IBD) and all the police resources (my immune system) are needed to help solve the murder. But at the same time there's lots of petty crime taking place (such as stress, not eating nutrient rich foods or late nights) and some of the police resources are being diverted to deal with the effects of this petty crime instead of being able to focus just on the murder (my IBD). So, by not having all the petty crime going on I can allow the police (aka my immune system) to focus all their energy on solving the murder.

"I'm able to join in normal social activities and have stopped even thinking about where toilets are"

What is a flare like for me now?

Firstly, let me explain that before I started working on improving my health my flares would be crippling. I would go to the toilet 30 times a day, see extreme amounts of blood in the toilet and feel tired constantly. Taking steroids would stop a flare within days, however if I dropped below 10mg I would deteriorate very quickly. I became completely steroid dependent and still needed to take them when I was on other medication.

Now, flares are a rarity. I have lots of energy, I go to the toilet once a day and my stools are formed. I hardly have any gas, no urgency to go to the toilet, my skin is clear and I am a stable weight. I'm able to join in normal social activities and have stopped even thinking about where toilets are. If I do need the toilet I'm able to hold on until I get to one.

I have become very intune with my body and can spot

---

a flare coming. The first signs of a decline in my health are depleted energy, tight muscles, being more gassy and having slightly less formed stools. When I feel these things happening I know I need to up my game and get more sleep, destress, eat better - whatever it is that is out of balance. Usually doing this brings me back into an equilibrium and the flare doesn't rear its ugly head. This can mean making some sacrifices in areas of my life for a few days. I may have to miss a night out or an event, be late for a deadline at work or not spend time with my wife and son. But, these short-term sacrifices can be the difference between curbing a flare or not, and being in a flare would mean making a lot more sacrifices for a longer period of time.

"Short-term sacrifices can be the difference between curbing a flare or not, and being in a flare would mean making a lot more sacrifices for a longer period of time"

On the rare occasions now that I can't get things quickly under control a flare involves being more gassy, having mucus in my stools which can progress to blood. Frequency and urgency to use the toilet will increase, I'll be more tired. During the worst flare I've had since coming off my medication, which was due to making people redundant at work, I was going to the toilet 10-15 times. This was when my calprotectin test results came back as 300. I was incredibly close to going back onto steroids to help me get back into remission. However, once I managed to get back in control of things (such as my stress) things started to improve and I was also able to get back into remission.

My day

On the next page I've included what a typical day looks like for me so you can see for yourself the things I do on a daily basis. Obviously everyday doesn't look exactly like this - things crop up which prevent me from always following this routine, but I try to stick to it as much as I possibly can.

The next chapter of this book delves in detail into these things and explains the theories behind why they may help me.

A lot of people tell me that they wouldn't have time to do all the things I do, and I completely understand that. I'm in a unique position that I can be quite flexible with my days due to having my own business. I also didn't introduce everything at once. I've started doing all of these things gradually over the past 6 years, adding a new thing in slowly so that it becomes a habit before moving onto the next thing. When I was very ill with my IBD I used to have up to 30 toilet trips a day and have to take a daily nap - this probably used to use up several hours of my time each day...time I didn't necessarily have but had no choice to find. Now, as my health has improved, I've needed less toilet trips and no naps so I've been able to use some of this time instead to focus on doing things for my health.

At the end of my typical weekday and weekend days you will also find some of the extra things I do when my health is deteriorating or I'm in a flare from my ulcerative colitis.

A typical weekday

6.30am

Woken up by my son. Stop the sleep tracking on my phone.

6.40am

Go downstairs. Take MSM. Toliet. Take Symprove. Start cooking breakfast.

7.10am

Eat breakfast - eggs, sweet potato, avocado, tomatoe and mushrooms. Drink cup of hot lemon and filtered water. Take supplements - magnesium glycinate, turmeric, colostrum, vitamin D.

7.30am

Shower with chemical free products, use natural deodorant and get dressed.

8.00am

Cycle/walk to work.

8.30am

Start work. Use my standing desk all day, drink filtered water as and when needed.

9.30am

Take short break (10mins). I usually do one of the following...

- Walk to beach
- Walk around the block, up and down the stairs - anywhere!
- Stretch
- Meditate
- Read book
- Light training/stretching

10.30am

Take short break.

11.30am

Take short break.

1.00pm-2.00pm

Lunch break. Go for a walk, sprint training, swim in sea, cycle or go to the gym. Eat lunch - fish or meat and vegetables/salad. Take supplements - magnesium glycinate, MSM, turmeric.

3.00pm

Take short break.

4.00pm

Take short break.

5.00pm

Finish work. Cycle/walk home.

5.15pm

Eat dinner - fish or meat and vegetables/salad, stew or tagine.

6.00pm

Bath son and put him to bed.

8.00pm

Stop using phone or watching TV. Put on blue light blocking glasses.

8.00pm

Go out on my bike, athletics training, listen to radio/podcast, do puzzle or have a sauna, do some gardening.

9.00pm

Spray magnesium oil on legs. Take supplements - magnesium, colostrum, melatonin. Do half an hour stretching.

9.30pm

Start sleep tracking. Go to sleep.

A typical weekend day

6.30am

Woken up by my son. Stop the sleep tracking on my phone.

6.40am

Go downstairs. Take Symprove. Take MSM. Start cooking breakfast.

7.10am

Eat breakfast - eggs, sweet potato, avocado, mushrooms and tomatoes. Drink cup of hot lemon and filtered water. Take supplements - magnesium glycinate, turmeric, colostrum, vitamin D.

7.30am

Play with son.

8.00am

Shower with chemical free products, use natural deodorant and get dressed.

8.30am

Help get son ready for the day.

9.30am

Go out somewhere with son - usually to a park, farm, beach, swimming.

12.30pm

Prepare and eat lunch - fish or meat and vegetables/salad. Take supplements - magnesium glycinate, MSM, turmeric.

1.30pm

Go out for walk with son - take him on his bike or scooter.

3.00pm

Play with son at home or in the garden.

5.30pm

Eat dinner - fish or meat and vegetables/salad, stew or tagine.

6.00pm

Bath son and put him to bed.

8.00pm

Stop using phone or watching TV. Put on blue light blocking glasses.

8.00pm

Go out on my bike, training, listen to radio/podcast, do puzzle or have a sauna.

9.00pm

Take supplements - magnesium, colostrum, melatonin. Do half an hour stretching.

9.30pm-10.00pm

Start sleep tracking. Go to sleep.

When I'm deteriorating

If I feel my health deteriorating I follow the routines above, but also try to add in some of the following things:

- Headspace (meditation app)
- Take it easy
- More strict with diet
- More strict with sleep
- Magnesium bath
- Nap
- Fasting
- Sauna

If I'm in a flare

If I'm in a flare I will also include the following things into my day. During a flare my health takes priority over anything else and I will cancel plans and take days off work to ensure that I recover as quickly as possible. I've found that if I don't do this I end up taking longer to recover and it impacts my life more in the longer term.

- Sleep till wake naturally
- Take day off work
- Walk
- Gentle exercise
- Meditate
- Eat well or do a bone broth fast
- Do enjoyable things (go cycling etc)
- Strict bedtime routine
- Sauna
- Magnesium bath

"I find that if I am hard on myself then it causes me stress and anxiety – and this isn't good for my health"

Discipline and willpower

It's worth adding a quick note here to say that I have days when I have incredibly strong willpower and discipline and don't stray from my routine. But, I also have days where I cave into temptation and will eat a whole bar of dark chocolate in one sitting or don't go for a run because it's cold and pouring with rain. On these days I try not to beat myself up and try to enjoy what I'm doing instead of following my routine. I find that if I am hard on myself then it causes me stress and anxiety – and this isn't good for my health (and it probably has a worse effect on me than the 'bad' thing I was doing in the first place). A treat or a late night now and then is fine, but if I find myself starting to do these on a frequent basis then I try to reign things in and instill a bit more discipline into my routine before my balance is upset. If I do stray too much then my body will soon give me signs that I need to be more disciplined.

Although it all seems like a lot of effort and hard work, and I've had to make some big sacrifices, I choose to live my life in this way. I'd much rather be doing all the things I do now than feel the way I did 5 years ago.

Practical living

On the following pages I will explain more about how and why I do some of the things I mention in my balance theory in the previous section.

I will cover the five elements of my 'balance theory'. These are:

- Mind & stress
- Sleep
- Diet & nutrition
- Movement & exercise
- Environment

Mind & stress management

I think stress is one of the biggest influencers on my health, and in turn my IBD. I run my own web design business, and have done since before I was diagnosed, and running your own company is full of stress.

One of the worst flares I have ever had was when I was making three staff redundant. Things got so bad I was hours from taking myself off to A&E to be admitted (and things have to be pretty bad for me to get to that point). But, somehow, I managed to pull through.

Stress comes in all sorts of different forms - it can be

physical, mental, emotional or chemical - but most of us are exposed to it in one form or another. It's how we learn to deal with it that's important. We have evolved to be able to cope with short bursts of stress (such as running away from a lion) and in the modern world a small amount of stress can be beneficial to help us finish a work project or get through an exam. But when that stress becomes chronic, in that it's there all the time, it can lead to problems.

"I think stress is one of the biggest influencers on my health, and in turn my IBD"

According to the NHS: "Stress is the feeling of being under too much mental or emotional pressure, and pressure turns into stress when you feel unable to cope. A bit of stress is normal and can help push you to do something new or difficult, but too much stress can take its toll."[1]

How stress affects the body

According to the American Psychological Association[2] "stress can make existing problems worse[3]. In one study, for example, about half the participants saw improvements in chronic headaches after learning how to stop the stress-producing habit of "catastrophizing", or constantly thinking negative thoughts about their pain.[4]"

I can certainly believe this and have found it with my own UC. Until only recently (and still sometimes now if my health has slipped) I struggled with urgency to use the toilet. And, the more I would stress - or 'catastrophize' - about what would happen if I didn't make it to the toilet the more I would need to go...until I would have an accident. Determined to break out of this cycle I started employing some techniques to help me, such as distracting myself with something (like a book or a game on my phone) or doing some deep breathing or meditation (I use an app, more on this later). At first it was hard, but the more times that I managed to make it to the toilet without soiling myself the more confident I became and the less stress I was placing on myself as a result. I can generally now 'hold on' for around 20 minutes (although I still do have occasions when I just can't wait but these are very few and far between).

Another study[5] found that 'chronic psychological stress is associated with the body losing its ability to regulate the inflammatory response' which could 'promote the development and progression of disease'[6].

Findings such as this led me to wonder if the reason I was finding stress so detrimental to my IBD was because it was preventing my body from controlling inflammation, which is known to cause IBD flares. Indeed, evidence is growing that psychological stress does "contribute to the risk of relapse in IBD"[7].

It has also been shown in mice that stress affects the structure of the intestinal microbiota[8]. Our gut microbiota (often referred to as our microbiome) is a collection of organisms that live in our intestinal tract. Researchers are now finding that these organisms have a huge influence over our well-being (or poor health). You can read more about the role the microbiome plays in the section about diet and nutrition.

Stress can lead to people losing sleep or becoming anxious or irritable. It can lead to people losing self-esteem, becoming angry or causing physical problems such as heart disease, asthma, stroke, diabetes and some types of cancer[9].

It can affect how you think, feel and behave. And, we have already seen above that it affects the body's inflammatory response and the risk of IBD relapses.

These can all have a dramatic effect on your quality of life.

What is the stress response (aka fight or flight)?

Stress is our body's biological or psychological response to a threat. When our body detects a threat it enters what we refer to as fight or flight mode. Historically we would enter this mode when we were facing a physical threat (such as being eaten by a lion). These acute episodes of fight or flight mode would help us either flee from the threat or stand up to it.

When we become stressed the hypothalamus (an area of the

brain that coordinates various systems in our body) sends signals to the pituitary gland (our body's master gland) and the adrenal medulla (which controls stress hormones). Once these signals have been received a cascade of hormones are released and our fight or flight response is triggered. At this point you may notice increased heart rate, slowing of digestion and increased energy and strength.

Although what is now perceived to be a threat has changed drastically, the fight or flight response is still incredibly important - but it may also be detrimental to our health if it is being triggered at the wrong times.

When faced with being hit by a car fight or flight mode can be important in saving us. However, in the modern world our stress response is being increasingly triggered more and more by things such as traffic jams, work deadlines or even just things we read in the news or see on social media.

It's thought that this constant activation of the stress response can take its toll on the body which is given no time to recover from the effects of the constant stream of stress hormones. This can result in heart issues, increased inflammation and even lead to chronic disease.

As mentioned earlier there are a few different types of stress we may find ourselves placed under, and sometimes you may not even realise your body is under stress.

Physical stress

You may be placed under physical stress by an illness or disease (such as IBD), intense exercise, working long hours, pregnancy.

Mental and/or emotional stress

You may be placed under mental or emotional stress through a bereavement, breakdown of a relationship, being unhappy in a job, being made redundant, becoming a parent, getting married, being a carer for a friend or family member, retiring, money worries, moving house, depression, anxiety, low self-esteem or other mental health issues.

Chemical stress

You may be placed under chemical stress through a food allergy or intolerance, medication you are taking, toxins you are exposed to.

How I manage stress

A few years ago I started really taking an interest in what stress was doing to my body, and more importantly what I could do to stop it having such negative effects.

I was getting headaches, feeling anxious, lying awake at night thinking about things, not being mentally present with my family and friends and a whole host of other symptoms that I didn't realise were being caused by stress until I started reducing it in my life.

We live in a fast-paced world and this can take its toll. Everyone expects everything instantly - replies to emails, news as it happens, online shopping delivered straight away. Our senses are constantly bombarded and are never given a moment to switch off. I don't think we talk, or do, enough about the stress we are all placed under. I see it all the time in fellow IBD patients I talk to - they are stressed and feel they can't cope but don't feel they can take some time out to recharge their batteries because of all the things they are expected to do, such as looking after children, excelling at work, maintaining friendships online and offline or running a household let alone living with IBD. It's hard. I was just as guilty (and still can be) so I knew that learning to deal with my stresses was going to be tough.

There were some things that were causing me (and my family) stress that I had known about for a long time but I had always tried to ignore them. But now was the time to really start to address them.

Before I could start work on reducing stress I needed to identify what the stressors actually were. I wrote these down so I was clear about them. Then I came up with some strategies to deal with them.

Here's what my list looked like in July 2016 and the ideas I came up with to help reduce some of these stressors:

Stressors	Solutions
Money - cash flow Running my own business means cash flow is an issue. People never pay on time and I am always having to try to win new web design work. This means I can't always be sure I can pay my staff or my mortgage. This situation is exacerbated by the fact that my wife, Emily, is employed by my business so we both rely on it for our income. I can't shut down the company and start again due to business debts in my name (see below)	• Find more regular sources of income • Reduce business and personal outgoings • Emily to get another job?
Money - business debts I have long-standing debts from when I first set up my business which I struggle to pay each month. Have previously been turned down for business loans	• Find a way to consolidate the debts or reduce payments

Stressors	Solutions
Working too much Having my own business, plus running IBDrelief.com means I put in a lot of hours. This causes me to not get as much sleep as I'd like and means I don't spend much time with my family	• Place working hours limits on myself • Add structured breaks into my working day (use Focus Keeper app to do this) • Block out time in my diary that I spend with my family
My health My UC is a constant worry. If I'm not in a flare I worry about when my next flare will be. I also get headaches and muscles pains which cause me stress	• Worry less! Start to meditate • Look at strategies to help reduce pain
My wife's health Emily has been suffering with poor health for a long time which no doctor has managed to get to the bottom of	• Be more forceful to get answers • Pay for private healthcare
DIY that needs finishing around the house Despite living in the house for several years there are still many jobs that I've left unfinished or haven't started. I get stressed whenever I look at something that isn't finished but don't have time to do it	• Lower my own expectations of what is possible • Finish the work • Pay someone to finish some of the work

Stressors	Solutions
Keeping on top of things around the house Due to both mine and my wife's poor health (and having a young child) we struggle to keep the house clean and tidy. This causes both of us stress	• Get a cleaner • Reduce expectations

The exercise of identifying all my stressors and solutions actually made me feel worse initially, not better. Seeing my problems written down and realising there were no quick fixes for any of them caused me a lot of anxiety for several weeks. But, after a while I came to terms with the fact that this was going to be a long journey and wasn't going to happen overnight. In fact it took me over a year-and-a-half to get to the point where I could honestly say my stress was largely under control.

Here's how I did it:

Money - cash flow

I knew I needed to be sure I was getting regular monthly payments into the business bank account. I began by starting to charge for some services that we were currently doing for free. I also identified some clients who would regularly come back for pieces of work and asked if they wanted to go on a monthly retainer. This way they would get a set number of hours of my time each month to use as they needed (and there would be a regular monthly direct debits into the business account from them). Some clients didn't want to do it, but several did. Emily started looking around for another job but as she needed to be part time (for childcare reasons) and due to her health we decided it wasn't the best course of action. We severely cut back on all costs - both personally and within the business. No more subscriptions to services, we changed utility providers, changed our mortgage, sublet a couple of rooms in our offices and made a member of staff redundant (which added to my short term stress but has now relieved a lot of it). The biggest change though was securing three days a week contractor work with one of my clients (and they pay on time each month!). It took around a year to do all this but the contract and the other changes meant all monthly outgoings were now nearly covered before I'd even taken on any other work.

Money - business debts

The debts had amounted over a few years when the company was first set up. There were several large debts owed to various different loan and credit card companies and many of them were in my name, so even if I declared the company bankrupt I would still be liable to pay them. The rates of interest on some of them were high. I was struggling to keep up the repayments. Several years before I'd tried to get a business loan to pay off all the debts and consolidate them into one place with a more manageable monthly payment. But, because the business wasn't making any money (due to paying off all the debts) no one would lend me the money. I'd previously avoided talking to my parents about the level of debt I was in (and the stress I was under) and hadn't even been honest about it with my wife. I knew though that now was the time for this to change. There were some difficult conversations (and quite a few tears) but they helped me to come up with some solutions. My parents took out a loan so I could pay off a large chunk of the credit cards and significantly reduce the monthly amount I was paying to cover the repayments. Emily's parents also lent me some money to cover some more of the debts and we took out a bigger mortgage when we renewed our deal to cover the rest. We were completely honest with our mortgage company about what we were going to do with the money and thankfully they saw the sense in it and agreed to lend us enough to cover the remaining amount. These three loans mean the monthly repayments have reduced significantly. I can't even describe to you what a huge weight has been lifted from my shoulders.

Working too much

Since setting up my business at 21 I've always known that I work too much. I think I believed that I wouldn't be successful if I didn't put in 60 hours a week and be contactable 24/7. It also became a habit - constantly checking work emails on my phone, working on my laptop in front of the TV in the evenings, staying in the office until 11pm each night to get a project finished. It was bad for my stress levels, bad for my health and bad for my personal relationships. I decided to place strict working hours on myself - Monday to Friday 8am-6pm and 9-1pm on a Saturday morning if I really needed to work some more. So, unless I had a big project on with a tight deadline I tried to stick to this. I turned off email notifications on my phone and everytime I found myself reading them outside of work hours I asked myself 'Is someone going to die or be seriously injured if I don't reply until the morning?'. The answer was always no and so I learnt to leave things until the following day. As yet, none of my clients have been critical of me for not responding straight away - in fact a few have even said they need to do the same and stop working in the evenings. I also started applying the pomodoro time management technique to my working day. The idea is that you break your day into small sections (such as 25 minutes in length) after working for this time you then take a short break (such as for 5 minutes) and then start the process again. Since starting this technique I've found I'm more focused and productive. I use an app called Focus Keeper to help with this. I've also had to reduce my own expectations on what I can achieve. When we set up IBDrelief we worked night and day to get it up and running and continue to add content to it. We had hoped to turn it into something that we could both work full time on and employ other people living with IBD too. But, we've had to readjust our expectations on this. For now I accept that my health is more impor-tant than burning myself into the ground to achieve it. Something else I did was block out a weekend a month for 'family time' - time I would just spend with my family. This helps me to feel better connected to them and is a time when I am completely focused on my little family and nothing else.

My health

If you have a condition which affects your life it's unusual not to worry about your health. I was certainly doing it a lot. Most of my concerns would centre around whether or not I'd be about to have a flare, but I'd also worry about the side effects of the medications I was taking, that my poor health was preventing me from doing things other people my age were doing or that my poor immune system would mean I'd catch yet another cold. I also worried about the future. 1 in 3 people with my condition (pan-ulcerative colitis) end up having surgery on their large intestine. Would that be me? And, I'm at a greater risk of developing bowel cancer. Then my consultant mentioned that I was also in a risk group for developing Primary Sclerosing Cholangitis (PSC), so would I develop that or one of the many other complications ulcerative colitis can cause? It was a never-ending cycle of worry and stress. Some people would tell me just not to think about it. But, how was I going to manage that? It's such a huge part of my life and not something you can just forget about. Plus, I feel it's important to have a degree of awareness about these things - I'm no longer the kind of person who can walk around in blissful ignorance. So, I decided I'd try meditating. Meditation is something I'd always thought was just for hippies but I'm now a complete convert. Firstly, I'd like to clarify that I don't do it sitting cross legged and chanting 'Om'. Sometimes I'm meditating and you wouldn't even know. I started by using an app (I used Headspace but there's plenty of other apps and online videos out there - I tried a few until I found one I liked). As a total beginner to meditation the app gave me a good introduction to how to do it and some useful techniques which I apply to my everyday life. Now I often find myself meditating without even realising, for example, when I'm sitting waiting for a train I'll count my breaths pass or as I'm walking somewhere I'll concentrate on the feeling of my feet touching the floor as I move. After meditating I feel a sense of calm and clarity come over me. So, if I find myself stressing about something I'll take a few minutes out just to do some breathing and I come away with a new perspective on the situation. It hasn't necessarily taken the worry away but it's changed how that worrying affects me.

My wife's health

For maybe 10 years Emily has struggled with various aspects of her health which no one in the NHS has been able to find the answers for. I could see that it was really starting to affect her mental health (she started to think it was all in her head even though there were some very real symptoms). I was, of course, worried about her and this worry was causing me to feel stressed. So, once I had sorted out my money issues I used some of the money that had been freed up to pay for her to see someone privately and get some testing done. It's been expensive, but so worth it as we are starting to get some answers. It's complicated and hard to manage but she's on the way to feeling a lot better (which is also making me feel better).

DIY

I enjoy doing DIY so when we moved into our house in 2011 I was excited that it needed a lot of work. And, despite my health I managed to do a lot of it myself. But, after 5 years there were still a lot of projects that needed doing or finishing. These would constantly play on my mind and I found myself getting quite down about the fact I hadn't been able to do them all, because I was too busy working or prioritising my health (and I also couldn't afford to pay someone else to do them). This caused me to become stressed about the outstanding tasks and I would think about them in the middle of the night. When this started to happen regularly I knew I needed to either get some of the work finished or lower my high expectations. I started by speaking to my wife about which jobs she felt were important that we got finished and focused my attention on those. Some of them we paid to have finished (using some of the money now being saved from sorting out my finances) but mostly I put time aside in my diary to get some of them done. Everytime I focused on the jobs that I hadn't managed to finish I applied the same principle that I did to my emails - I'd ask myself if someone was going to die or be injured as a result of the DIY not being finished. A lot of the jobs were just cosmetic and it helped me to put them into perspective. However, I still struggle with this as the list seems to constantly be growing as I get other jobs done!

Housework

Seeing piles of dishes and dust everywhere and knowing that the bathroom or kitchen hadn't been cleaned for several weeks would stress me out. We'd talked about getting a cleaner for years but never thought we could justify the cost. We thought we'd soon find the time or feel better enough to do it ourselves - why pay someone to do a job you could do yourself, right? Except we couldn't and didn't do it ourselves. So, about a year ago we bit the bullet and got a cleaner. I wish we had done it so much sooner. Every Monday we get home from work and the house is clean and tidy. Our home has changed from being a stressful place to spend time in to a positive environment. Having a nice, clean space to spend time does wonders for your mood and stress levels and takes a weight off your mind. I'd highly recommend it!

Mental health

I'm lucky that my mental health has never been severely affected from living with IBD. Looking back retrospectively at the times when my IBD was at its worst I definitely did have some struggles though. My main issues were coping with stress (as discussed above) and anxiety. My anxiety would mostly be related to my disease - anxiety about finding a toilet, anxiety about soiling myself, embarrassment about some of the symptoms of the disease (such as passing a lot of wind) and anxiety about having to get up in the middle of a meeting or meal to go and use the toilet. At times I would sit on the toilet and cry, angry and frustrated.

As my disease has improved, this anxiety has moved into the background and I'm able to go about my life without having to really think about a lot of these things.

But, I know that this isn't the case for many people - and it's completely understandable. Having a chronic condition like IBD is life-changing and affects everyone in such different ways. I'm also not complacent. I know that just because my mental health is ok now, doesn't mean it will always remain that way.

To keep myself in a good place I try to make sure I do something fun on a daily basis. For me that means going out cycling or for a run, watching football or playing games or tickling my son until he can't laugh anymore. I find this is really important to also reduce my stress levels.

I've never really spoken to anyone independent, such as a counsellor, about my disease and the effect it has had on my life. I'm certainly open to the idea of doing this though and is something I may try in the future if I feel I need to.

My mind and stress takeaways

Here's a summary of the things I've done to help combat my stresses...

- Mindfulness and meditation - there are some great apps out there which supported me to get started. I personally use Headspace and now don't even need to use it to do a 10-15 minute practise.

- Outsource tasks - I outsourced tasks that other people could help with, (such as cleaning).

- Lower expectations - this is a hard thing to do but over time I gradually let go of expectations more and more

- Identify what stressed me out and then face them head on - this was painful in the short time but better in the long run.

- Put aside time to do enjoyable things - I schedule them into my diary and do them!

- Work less - not achievable for everyone, but I was able to cut down my hours.

- Don't take work home - many of us do it, either physically or emotionally, and I'm very guilty of it. I've learnt to leave work at work.

- Make time to have some fun.

Sleep

The amount and quality of sleep I get is another big influencer on my IBD. It used to be that if I had a rough night I could almost guarantee I would spend the following day on the toilet. My fatigue would also be high and for a few years after my diagnosis I would find myself needing to go home at lunchtime to take a nap (I was lucky that owning my own business meant I could do this). Thankfully, now that my general health is in a better place, I can get away with one or two bad nights. But, if these start to add up then my health seriously suffers.

I feel that more and more humans are placing less emphasis on the importance of sleep for everyone, not just those of us living with health conditions, despite research continually pointing out the dangers insufficient sleep can have to our health. In today's world there are far too many temptations to stay up beyond our bedtime binge watching box sets, scrolling through social media into the early hours or even doing your weekly grocery shop at 3am. It almost seems like a competition to see who can survive on the least amount of sleep. Going to bed early just isn't cool. But, it's not just the time that we go to bed that's the problem. Insomnia and disturbed sleep are an increasing problem for many, meaning that even if they go to bed early they just aren't getting the quality of sleep that's needed to maintain good health.

What is the circadian rhythm?

The body's internal clock works primarily on how much dark and light we are exposed to. When we are exposed to large amounts of light the body thinks it's daytime and as this light decreases the body starts to get ready for sleep. This is known as our circadian rhythm. This worked fine when our only source of light was the sun. However, now we are not exposed to enough natural light in the day, particularly in the morning, and then to many sources of artificial light in the evening/at night (such as TVs and our mobile phones) which throws our circadian rhythm out of time. Not only does the circadian rhythm control when we want to wake and sleep it also controls other physiological processes in our body such as when we want to eat, brain activity, hormone production and cell regeneration.

We can help readjust this by increasing our exposure to natural light in the mornings and making sure we reduce the amount of light exposure in the evenings and at night.

Why do we need sleep?

Sleep is how our body recoups energy. During sleep our brain stores memories from the day and it helps our mental and emotional wellbeing to be restored. There's a reason

"It would be the biggest evolutionary mistake if sleep does not serve some critical function"

we are often told to "sleep on it" when we need to make a difficult decision or are facing hard times. It's also a time our body builds and repairs itself and boosts your immune system.

A lack of sleep has been linked to an increased risk of death[10]. It's also linked to increased obesity[11] and increased inflammation[12]. There's also studies which suggest that increased inflammation in your body can actually cause sleep disturbances[13] - meaning you could end up in a vicious cycle of needing sleep to reduce inflammation but not being able to get any because of inflammation.

As Matthew Walker, director of the Sleep and Neuroimaging Lab at the University of California, Berkley, says: "It would be the biggest evolutionary mistake if sleep does not serve some critical function."[14]

How I increased the quality of my sleep

After realising the amount and quality of sleep I was getting correlated to how my body and health felt I decided I wanted to try to optimise it as much as possible. The first thing I did was to download a sleep tracker (I use SleepCycle) onto my phone so I could start to get a truer picture of what my sleep was like. After a few weeks this started to give me some insights into my sleep.

Although I was going to bed around 10.30pm and waking at 6.30am (so in bed for 8 hours) I was still waking up feeling tired. The app helped me to realise that I wasn't getting the quality of sleep I needed, even though I may have been getting the quantity. The thing I really like about the SleepCycle app is that it gives a simple % quality score for your night's sleep. When I started using it although I was getting over 8 hours' sleep my quality score was between 50-60%. I couldn't believe that I was losing out on over 40% of quality sleep. How great could I feel if I could get to 70,80 or even 90%? Over time I have worked on the quality of my sleep (more to follow) and I now regularly get over 90% - on some occasions I have even reached 100%!

It used to take me quite a while to fall asleep (maybe half an hour or so) and I would wake several times in the night. Sometimes this would be to use toilet (if my IBD wasn't in a good place), sometimes because my wife was awake (she's not a very good sleeper!), sometimes because my son had woken and sometimes for unexplained reasons. On many occasions it would then take me another half hour or so to get settled again. This meant that in a night where I would wake twice I was losing an hour-and-a-half's sleep just trying to get to sleep.

The tracker also showed me I wasn't getting as much deep sleep as I probably should be. Although the quality of information in these trackers isn't completely accurate, it gave me an indication I wasn't going through a full sleep cycle to aid recovery etc. I'm now very in tune with how my body feels and I can certainly notice the difference if my sleep quality decreases, particularly over a period of time.

Not only do I find tracking my sleep as a good indication of how well I'm sleeping but I also now use it as a way of indicating how good my overall health is. If I see a decline in my sleep quality (and it's not for an obvious reason, such as a late night) it could be because I'm experiencing an increase in stress I hadn't been aware of or I haven't been doing enough exercise. Often this is one of the first indications I have (before the toilet symptoms start) that my health is declining and my IBD may be coming into a flare.

The 4 stages of sleep

When we are sleeping we go through sleep cycles. Each cycle typically lasts between 90-120 minutes - so during a night we may go through four or five cycles. Each sleep cycle consists of 4 stages.

NREM stage one (light sleep)
This stage happens just after you close your eyes. You are lightly asleep and can go back to being awake very quickly. You may experience muscle twitching and a sense of falling during this stage. It typically lasts between 1-10 minutes.

NREM stage two (light sleep)
This stage is still considered as light sleep but it becomes harder to wake you. Your heart rate slows, your body temperature decreases, as does your blood pressure and other metabolic functions slow down.

NREM stage 3 (deep sleep)

You tend to fall into this stage around 35-45 minutes after going to sleep. Your brain waves slow down and you can sleep through most disturbances. If you are woken during this stage of sleep you will probably feel disorientated.

REM stage 4 (deep sleep)

During the final stage of a sleep cycle you enter REM - rapid eye movement - sleep (yes, your eyes do move rapidly). This is the deepest stage of sleep and where our dreams usually happen. During the first sleep cycle this stage usually only lasts for around 10 minutes, but as the night goes on it gets longer and can last up to an hour by the end of the night. Deep sleep provides the most restorative rest. During deep sleep the body repairs muscles and tissues, carries out growth and development, boosts immune function and gathers energy for the following day.

Now that I knew my sleep wasn't as good as it could have been, despite spending 8 hours a night in bed, I needed to figure out how to fix it. I started by reading lots of articles by sleep experts talking about how to improve sleep quality. At the same time I also moved my bedtime forward to 9.30pm to try to counteract the time I was losing trying to get to sleep. My aim was to get 8 hours of quality sleep a night. For me the focus is always on quality, not quantity. I've noticed that if I 'prepare' properly for sleep in the hours running up to bedtime (such as reducing bluelight, having a sleep routine - more on these to follow) I can get better quality sleep. Straight away I noticed a difference in my earlier bedtime, I had less fatigue during the day and was needing to nap less frequently.

Here is an example of when I first used the app in 2016. Although I got 8:28 hours' sleep my score was 61%. Since then I've found that when I wake up early in the night (around midnight-1am) this has a negative effect on the sleep score I get.

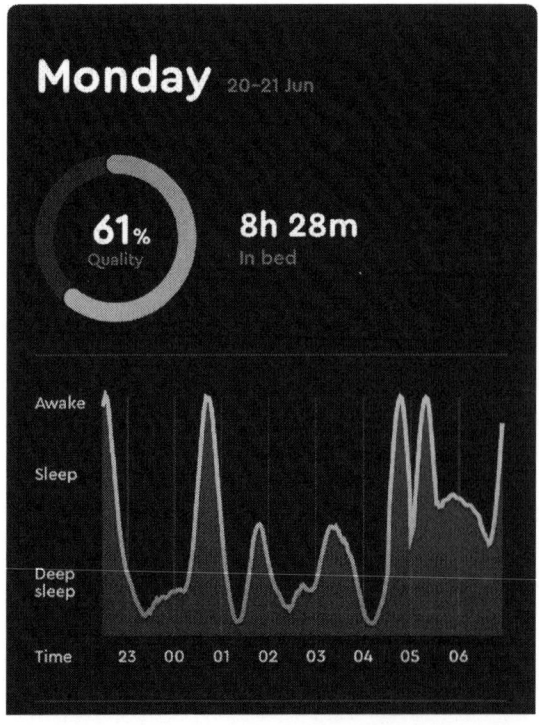

Only 60% sleep quality, despite over eight hours sleep

Below is an example of when I had a longer sleep (10:25 hours) which actually didn't give me an amazing sleep score - showing that quality is better than quantity! I also woke quite a few times during the night so perhaps I just wasn't tired enough.

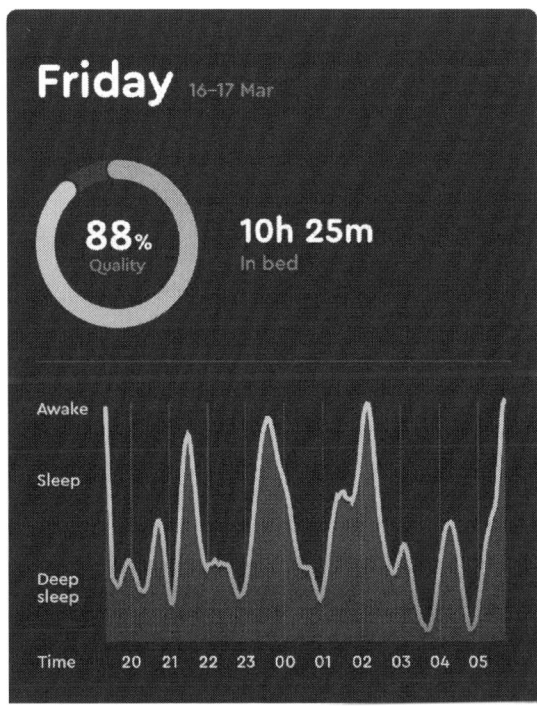

Despite a longer sleep I didn't reach 100%

There are times now when I get a near perfect sleep score (and on a couple of occasions I've even managed to get 100%). These seem to happen when I get a few hours of undisturbed deep sleep at the beginning of the night and am able to wake up naturally without being woken by my alarm or my son.

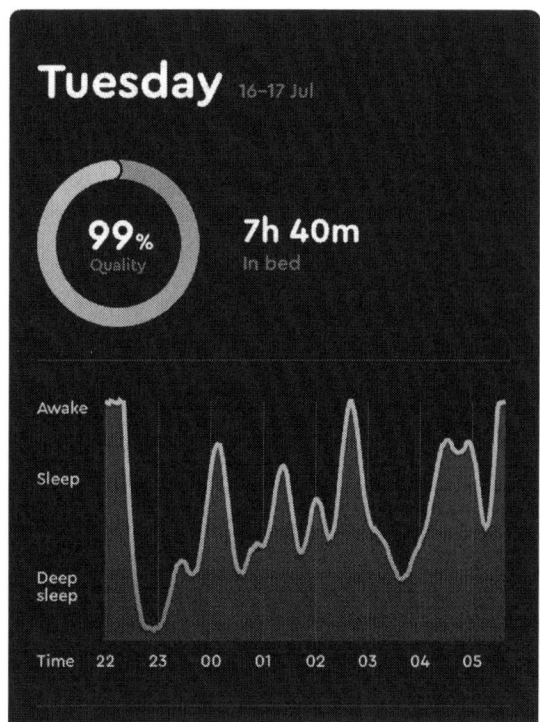

Tuesday 16–17 Jul

99% Quality

7h 40m In bed

Awake

Sleep

Deep sleep

Time 22 23 00 01 02 03 04 05

Good amount of undisturbed sleep early on resulting in high sleep score (despite shorter time in bed)

Now that I've been using the SleepCycle app for a while I've been able to build up a picture of what particular things affect my sleep the most, with my son being awake in the night ill and alcohol affecting my sleep quality the most.

Decreased sleep quality

-24%	Hayden up in night
-24%	Hayden ill
-13%	Ate late
-10%	Hot
-9%	Alcohol
-7%	Tv
-4%	Worked late
-2%	Cooler
-1%	Stressful day

Causes of decreased sleep quality

I'm also able to see what my sleep quality looks like over a period of time. It has allowed me to see that when my IBD symptoms aren't very good my sleep quality decreases. For example, there were drops in March/April in 2018 when I was feeling particularly stressed and was on the edge of a flare up and a bigger decrease in June/July 2018 when the weather was hot so I wasn't sleeping and my son was very ill for a couple of weeks causing me to awake in the night. During this time my symptoms did start to show, but I didn't reach the point of a flare as I worked very hard at restarting my balance.

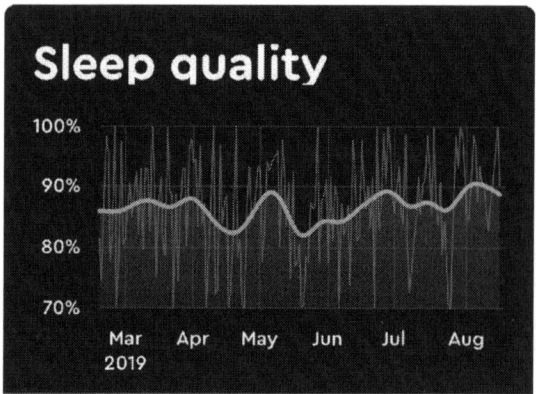

Sleep quality over time

Learning more about sleep also led me to make lots of little changes (I've gone into more detail about below) which helped to improve the quality of the sleep I was getting. Two years on from starting to track my sleep I now feel great day-to-day. I can't remember the last time I needed to nap (apart from when I've had a bad cold) and I'm able to concentrate throughout the day without needing stimulants, such as sugar and caffeine to give me a boost.

Here, and in no particular order, are some of the other changes I made...

Reduce blue light

Blue light is emitted by electronic devices (such as computers, televisions, phones, tablets and backlit e-readers) and energy-efficient lightbulbs. It's everywhere in our modern world, but more and more research is showing that blue light can be harmful to our health, especially when we are exposed to it at night time.

How does blue light affect sleep?

The wavelengths produced by blue light boost attention, reaction time and mood[15]. This is great news during the day, but bad news when we are trying to wind down to sleep in the evenings. Naturally we receive blue light from the sun during the day, but when the sun goes down our exposure to blue light is reduced.

However, as we are now using more and more devices which emit blue light in the evenings we are disrupting this natural cycle. Blue light has been shown to reduce the release of the hormone melatonin which helps to control your sleep and wake cycles.

Melatonin starts to be released a couple of hours before you go to sleep (at the time when blue light from the sun naturally starts to drop) and peaks in the middle of the night. When devices which emit blue light are used during this time melatonin production is delayed, meaning we don't feel sleepy until later, thus delaying the time we go to bed and disrupting our sleep-wake cycle.

Exposure to blue light in the evenings can disrupt our circadian rhythm making our bodies think that it's the middle of the day (see info box on blue light). Watching TV, scrolling through social media on your phone, using your laptop to check your emails are activities that we are all guilty of in the evenings.

Once I began to learn about the damaging effects blue light can have on sleep I started to become more aware of the exposure to it I was getting in the hours leading up to bed. I'd regularly sit and watch a football game on TV, while doing some work on my laptop or interacting with people on social media. I'd also have all the lights in the house on full blast so that I could see what I was doing. All of these were exposing me to a huge amount of blue light, but breaking out of these long-lived habits was hard. To help I removed notifications for social media and emails from my phone so I was less tempted to check these. I also introduced a rule that I wasn't to use any electronic devices in the 90 minutes before I was going to bed. With my new bedtime of 9.30pm this meant that from 8pm I had to switch off the TV and my laptop and stop checking my phone. It also meant I had to find other activities to occupy my time so I wasn't tempted to check Facebook. My son tends to be in bed by 6pm, so putting him to bed at this time re-minds me I need to stop using screens (and I follow the same rule for him - no more CBeebies after dinner!). I started doing puzzles, listening to music, the radio and podcasts...and started spending time talking to other people, either on the phone or in person, in the eve-nings! I bought some blue light blocking glasses so that the blue light I was still exposed to (such as lights around the house) or the occasional text message was minimised. I also now use f.lux on my laptop and Night Shift mode on my phone which both lower the amount of blue light emitted.

I quickly found that by reducing my blue light exposure I was dropping off to sleep quicker and was having less un-explained awakenings in the night. Now I definitely notice a difference if I have to work on my laptop late or decide to watch a football game on TV. If I have been exposed to blue light in the evenings rather than jumping straight into bed after switching off the TV/laptop I'll spend 45 minutes or so unwinding - maybe doing some stretching or having a bath.

Improve my sleep routine

The times I went to bed and got up during the week were pretty consistent but at weekends I would often stay up later in the evenings and was still being woken at 6.30am by my son. So, I started going to bed at the same time at the weekends as I did in the week. Luckily (or unluckily) since having a child my social life has taken a dip and it's rare now that I go out on a Friday or Saturday night. If I do and don't get to bed until late I try not to beat myself up about it but I do try to make sure I don't do too much the day after and that I get to bed early the following evening. Since doing this I feel like I have more energy at weekends and get less headaches.

Increase movement during the day

I've always been a very active person but I would often have days when the only times I would move would be to go to and from the toilet at work. During my research into sleep I kept reading about the importance of doing movement during the day to improve the quality of sleep. One study found that people sleep better and feel more alert during the day if they get at least 150 minutes of exercise a week[16].

I certainly noticed this from the SleepCycle app - generally the more activity I do the greater increase in sleep quality I get.

"People sleep better and feel more alert during the day if they get at least 150 minutes of exercise a week"

Once I read this I started to notice that on days when I'd been very sedentary I wouldn't feel as refreshed in the morning. So, I started to make a conscious effort to move more. This didn't mean going for a run every day but meant increasing the amount of time I spent moving about. I did this by going for a walk during my lunch break a couple of times a week, forcing myself to get up from my desk every hour and do some stretches or walk to the toilet or kitchen. More recently I bought a standing desk for my office which means I now spend most of my day standing up. It's amazing how much more I move about now - maybe sitting at my desk was a barrier to moving. I also have a fitness tracker watch which counts my steps and, although I don't think it's truly accurate, it does give me a good

I pull it back and focus on my breath again (this is a technique I've learnt from the Headspace app). Another technique I use is to try to envisage going somewhere, such as walking to my office. I picture getting out of bed, walking down the stairs, putting on my shoes and coat, leaving the house, walking down the street. I try to picture every step, every last detail. If I get distracted by thinking of something else I start again. I've never made it much further than my front door before falling asleep!

Improve sleep hygiene

Sleep hygiene isn't about how clean we are when we are sleeping but about the habits and practices that we adopt to help us sleep better.

Things such as a dark, quiet room which isn't too hot can make a big difference to the quality of the sleep we get. One study got participants to sleep with a light on all night and then sleep without any light. It found "sleeping with the light on not only causes shallow sleep and frequent arousals but also has a persistent effect on brain oscillations, especially those implicated in sleep depth and stability"[17].

A 2018 study also found that exposure to even low levels of light while sleeping can lead to depressive symptoms[18].

I've had blackout blinds on my windows for several years but they don't make the room as dark as I'd like so I started wearing an eye mask. I didn't get on with the first sleep mask I used but I've now found one - a Manta sleep mask - that I find much more comfortable. I don't use it every night, but just when I feel I need to. I'm currently looking at getting a better quality blackout blind so that I don't have to use a sleep mask at all.

I've also experimented with using ear plugs to block out sound. This isn't always practical for me to do though as I often need to be able to hear if my son wakes in the night.

Over the years I've bought countless pillows to find one that I'm most comfortable with. It's taken a while but I'm finally happy with one and whenever I go away I always try to take it with me. I also use another two pillows to get myself into a comfortable sleeping position. I sleep on my right hand side and have one pillow between my knees and I 'cuddle' the other pillow. If I don't do this I find I get painful legs and arms where the knees and elbows meet each other. The mattress I sleep on is also important. By sheer luck we found a memory foam mattress (Simba) a few years ago that both my wife and I were instantly happy with. We've never stayed anywhere that has one as comfortable as ours.

I've already mentioned that I now go to bed and get up at the same time most days. This is another important part of my sleep hygiene. In the run up to my bedtime I also now do a relaxing activity. The activity I do varies from day-to-day depending on how I'm feeling and how much time I have, but can include light stretching, having a bath with epsom salts/magnesium, a sauna (I'm lucky enough to have one in my house), some meditation or doing a puzzle. This helps me to 'wind down' after the day and ensures I'm not thinking about anything stressful before going to bed.

Dietary changes

The things we eat and drink can play a part in the quality of our sleep at night. It's widely known that stimulants, such as caffeine, can negatively affect our sleep[19]. And, although alcohol may help some people to fall asleep faster, it can affect your quality of sleep later in the night[20] as your body processes the alcohol.

Because of this it's important to avoid caffeinated drinks - such as tea, coffee and energy drinks - and alcohol close to bedtime (some studies suggest avoiding caffeine up to 6 hours before bed[21]). I've never been a big drinker of either caffeine or alcohol so I didn't need to make too many changes in this area.

However, after my son was born in 2015 the time I would eat my dinner became later and later due to commitments with putting him to bed or working in the evenings. After getting him to sleep I would often find it was getting quite late and I'd have my dinner and then go straight to bed myself. I found this uncomfortable as my body digested the food. So, I decided to make a big shift in my evening routine and start eating dinner before my son went to bed. This meant dinner would need to be on the table by 6.30pm each night. At first my wife and I found it hard to fit cooking dinner into our routine. It didn't leave us long between getting home from work and needing to eat. It also meant we missed out on spending some time with our son who we hadn't seen all day. So, we started doing some prep on a Sunday evening for the week ahead which meant meals were quicker to put together Monday to Friday. We would do things such as roasting a chicken and lots of vegetables so that we had enough to last us for a couple of meals. We'd also make a big batch of a lamb tagine or stew and freeze portions. Doing this meant meals would always take under 15 minutes to prepare. We'd also make lots of stir frys which were quick and easy to throw together. By the time my 9.30pm bedtime had come my food had been given 3 hours to start digesting (instead of the hour or less it previously had). This also had the added bonus of giving me at least a 12 hour fasting period between my dinner and breakfast. You can read more about fasting in the section on diet and nutrition.

To aid with my sleep I also started taking a few supplements - magnesium, vitamin D and melatonin.

Magnesium

Magnesium helps to relax muscles and decrease cortisol[22] (the 'stress hormone'). Studies also suggest that it 'may have a role in the modulation of sleep quality'[23].

I started off using a magnesium spray on my muscles (mostly my legs) to help relax them before going to bed. I found I was often waking in the night because my muscles were tight. This helped to stop this happening. More recently I've started taking oral magnesium supplements.

Magnesium has a laxative effect if taken orally so I avoid it if I'm in a flare and just use a topical magnesium spray.

Vitamin D

Vitamin D is known as the 'sunshine' vitamin as our body produces it after exposure to the sun. It's estimated that between 30-50% of people are deficient in vitamin D[24]. Research has started to indicate that vitamin D may influence sleep quality and quantity[25]. Following a blood test which showed I was low on vitamin D levels I started taking an oral spray supplement. I take it in the morning after brushing my teeth. This mimics the effects of morning sun exposure on my skin. Vitamin D is also a powerful anti-inflammatory - so taking the supplement is a win-win for me! You can read more about vitamin D in the section on diet and nutrition later in this book.

Melatonin and sleep

Melatonin is produced naturally in our bodies and is responsible for telling us that it's time to go sleep. It also helps control our sleep-wake cycle. But melatonin production can be disrupted by exposure to light in the evenings (as mentioned earlier). I now take a melatonin supplement in the evenings to help boost my levels of this important sleep hormone. Melatonin has the added bonus of being anti-inflammatory[26] and helps relieve GERD and heartburn[27].

Improve wife's sleep

Whatever I did to improve my sleep didn't matter though if my wife's sleep was poor, causing me to be disturbed during the night. Although she drops off to sleep very easily (it often only takes her 5 minutes or less) she has always struggled with staying asleep throughout the night. She gets up at least twice, if not more, to use the toilet and then finds it difficult to get comfortable again. To help she has started using all the techniques I now use to improve her sleep. One of the things she has found most useful is wearing an eye mask to make sure light isn't disturbing her. Her sleep has improved greatly, but there are still periods where she struggles and during these times I do find myself heading off to the spare room so that my own sleep (and health) isn't compromised! I'll also proactively often sleep alone if I'm in a flare, under stress or know that my sleep is going to be affected by something else.

My sleep now

My sleep has improved greatly since I first started focusing on it nearly two years ago. During this whole time I've used the same sleep tracking app. At first I was receiving sleep quality marks of around 50% (or less) but now I regularly see over 80%. I use this sleep percentage as a loose predictor for what my health is going to be like. My health can cope with a couple of nights under 70% but if I drop below this amount for a sustained period (such as over a week) I know that my health is going to suffer. If I do start to see a decline I analyse why this might be and try to change it because I know that otherwise my health will be affected. I try to work out why my sleep might be poor. I consider whether I'm ill, stressed or in pain. Sometimes it might be because my son is unwell and waking frequently. Once I've identified the reason I consider what I can do to improve my sleep or mitigate against the effect of having some bad nights' sleep by doing more things from my 'good' side in my balance theory (see 'My balance theory' section).

Here is an example of what my sleep usually looks like if I follow a 'good' sleep routine before bed - I get lots of quality deep sleep early on in the night.

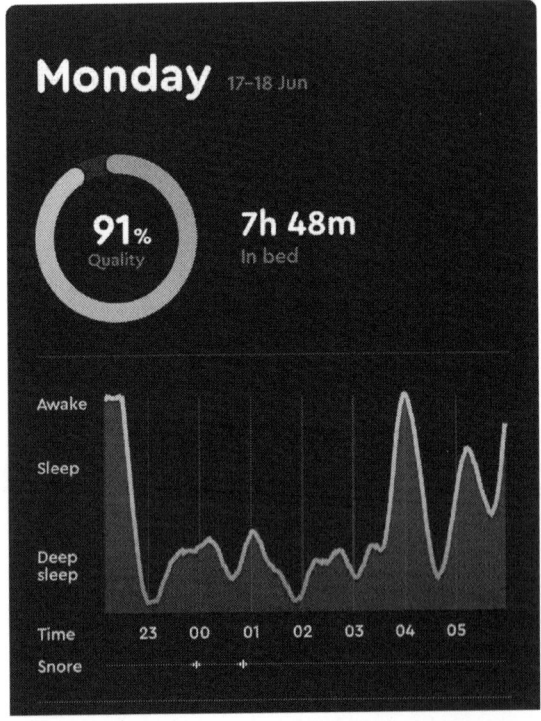

Monday 17–18 Jun

91% Quality   **7h 48m** In bed

Awake

Sleep

Deep sleep

Time   23   00   01   02   03   04   05

Snore

Deep sleep early on in the night usually gives me a high sleep quality score

indication as to whether I've spent the day being sedentary
or not. I'm quite a competitive person so I do regularly find
myself trying to beat my previous day's steps!

Get outside

Learning more about our circadian rhythm (see info box
earlier in this section) made me realise I needed to make
sure my body was aware when it was daytime and when
it was night. Reducing blue light in the evenings helped
me with the latter. So, to help my body realise it was day
I decided to try to get outside into natural light every
morning. By exposing myself to some sunlight first thing
I'm kick-starting my circadian rhythm and letting my
body know that's it's morning. During the week this is
quite easy as I either walk or cycle to work but at weekends
I have to try harder. Sometimes I really don't feel like it,
but even just taking 10 minutes in the morning to go for
a quick walk in the rain can make a huge difference to my
energy levels and alertness.

Reduce stress

I've gone into more details elsewhere in this book about
how I've reduced stress in my life and the benefits of doing
so. One of these has most definitely been an improvement
in my sleep. Now when I go to bed my head is a lot clearer
and thoughts don't invade my mind as I'm trying to drift
off. Of course, I still have nights when I struggle. If I'm
having one of these then I try counting my breaths - odd
numbers for in breaths, even for out. When I reach 10 I
start back at 1 again. If my mind drifts away from counting

My sleep takeaways

Here's a summary of the things I've done to support better sleep...

- Track sleep - use a sleep tracker on phone or a wearable watch to see what sleep cycles look like. Although not perfect this gives an indication as to any periods of time spent awake or if I'm not getting enough deep sleep

- Get regular time in bed. I try to go to bed and get up at the same time everyday. Aim for at least 8 hours in bed

- Reduce blue light. I cut out use of electronic devices 90 minutes before bedtime and lower lighting levels

- Use breathing techniques for the times when I can't get to sleep

- Move more - increase movement during the day. This could just be going for a walk in my lunch break and getting up from my desk or sofa at regular intervals to do some stretching

- Get outside - I try to get outside into natural light every morning

- Limit caffeine and alcohol before bed

- Eat earlier - I try to eat around 6.30pm

- Supplement with magnesium, vitamin D and melatonin

- Improve wife's sleep (or sleep in the spare room!)

Diet and nutrition

The topic of food and IBD is often talked about and greatly debated by both medical professionals and patients. There is no scientific evidence of specific diets that help IBD but many patients often avoid a great list of foods (or even whole food groups) they feel affect them. And, I'm no different. But, over the years the food I eat (and don't eat) has changed dramatically.

"I was very fatigued and would constantly be looking to consume as many calories as possible to give me energy"

When I was first diagnosed I survived for several years on a diet of Haribo sweets, cakes, biscuits, bread, packaged sandwiches, pizza and white potatoes (mainly in the form of chips). It doesn't take much to realise this was not going to be providing my body with the nutrition it needed to function, let alone support it to fight my IBD. But, back then didn't really think about this. I chose this diet partly because I was told by a gastroenterologist that fibre was bad for me and I should avoid it, and partly because I'd read negative experiences from other people with IBD in relation to fibre. I also used to make food choices based on the number of calories contained in them. I was very fatigued and would constantly be looking to consume as many calories as possible to give me energy. I felt I was an active person and that, combined with the many toilet trips I was making, would mean I wasn't going to put on weight.

"I search out nutrient-dense food to nourish my body and support it to be the strongest version of itself it possibly can be"

This view is not one I hold any more. Although I still no longer care about the number of calories I consume I don't go out of my way to seek them. Instead I search out nutrient-dense food to nourish my body and support it to be the strongest version of itself it possibly can be. For several years a fruit or vegetable hardly passed my lips. Today there isn't one I don't eat and sugar is a very rare treat that I enjoy, not something I survive on for hourly energy. But, it's taken me a long time to get to a place where I am able to do this. There were a lot of mental and physical barriers for me to overcome around my food choices. The most important part of this has been educating myself better about what our bodies need in order to thrive and fight disease and inflammation.

What is nutrition?

Nutrition is all about providing our bodies with the nutrients necessary for our health and growth. Our body needs certain nutrients to carry out various functions which are vital for our survival. If we aren't getting the right nutrition then this can lead to malnutrition and seriously damage our health. Malnutrition in IBD patients can also be caused by our body's inability to absorb nutrients from the food we are eating due to damage in the gastrointestinal tract caused by the disease.

In my case I think I mostly wasn't getting the nutrients

I needed because I wasn't eating enough of them. But I was probably also struggling to absorb the nutrients I was eating because of damage in my gut. At this time I found myself suffering from serious fatigue, headaches, iron deficiency and generally feeling unwell. I can't directly correlate these symptoms to my diet at the time, but since I've started eating more nutrients and fibre I feel a lot better.

The first time I really thought about changing my diet was when I went to visit a family friend who was an acupuncturist (you can read more about this in the 'My story' section). He suggested I stop eating gluten, dairy, sugar and nightshades (tomatoes, potatoes, aubergines, peppers). Advice like this wasn't usually something I would entertain. I'd been told by countless well-meaning people that I should change my diet, I should eat turmeric, I should try aloe vera, had I tried juicing? However, this time I was really struggling with my health and I just decided to give it a go.

I thought that if I cut out these foods and it didn't work I could easily reintroduce them again. So I started the following day and after a few weeks, to my complete surprise, I felt so much better. The process of cutting out these foods forced me to start to analyse the food I was eating. I knew that carrots and sweet potatoes (my orange diet as my wife called it) were safe for me so I started eating more of these. I also introduced some other similar root vegetables (such as butternut squash and parsnip). Instead of bread I switched to a gluten and dairy free version and I cut out the cakes and sweets I was living off of. I also ate more apples and bananas. As I (and my wife) got more and more used to catering for this new diet (and I started to feel some improvements in my symptoms) I experimented more with introducing other foods and cutting back on the amount of processed gluten and dairy free foods I was eating as I knew these foods were bad for me.

The best thing I did was to introduce a daily homemade smoothie to increase my vegetable and fibre intake. This had the added bonus of feeding my gut microbiome (learn more about this a bit later in this chapter). My recipe varied each day but it would generally include a few of the following: kale, spinach, cucumber, avocado, courgette, carrot and a piece of fruit, such as a banana or apple. Granted, it didn't taste great - but it wasn't about the taste. I viewed it the same as bad tasting medicine - something that you just had to put up with. By completely blending all the fruit and vegetables my body didn't need to do this work meaning they were easier to digest. At first I peeled all the fruit and veg but as I got more confident I started to leave the skins on as they contain a lot of nutrients.

Eventually I was able to re-introduce salad leaves and seeds (which I'd always avoided after seeing them in the toilet during a flare - more on this later) to my diet and now it's mainly just gluten and dairy I completely avoid and I minimise sugar and processed foods.

Gluten and dairy free foods

My View: When I first went gluten and dairy free I used to raid the 'free from' aisle in the supermarket looking for alternatives to the bread, cakes, pizza bases and cheese I could no longer eat. The majority of these products were nothing like the originals - but some of them were not too bad. However, I quickly realised that many of these 'free from' foods were ultra-processed, packed full of sugar and flavourings and many ingredients I'd never heard of. Because of this, and as I became more confident in catering for my new diet, I made a conscious effort to gradually phase a lot of them out. These products were great to get me started to make changes to my diet but now I will only eat them occasionally or if I'm in a restaurant and there is no alternative. I find I no longer crave these foods and much more enjoy the tastes and flavours of all the vegetables, fruits, herbs and spices I now use rather than trying to replicate my old diet. People seem to forget that if you are gluten and/or dairy free you don't need to just eat 'free from' foods. All vegetables, fruit, unprocessed meat, fish, herbs, nuts and seeds are naturally gluten and dairy free. This gave me a huge range of food options and exciting flavours to choose from.

As I started to notice an improvement in my symptoms (less toilet trips, less bloating) I wanted to learn more about why changing my diet could be helping. I started reading lots of research papers into diet and nutrition - not just those focusing on IBD but also on other autoimmune diseases, inflammation and general health and wellbeing. My reading quickly led me to discover the importance of our gut microbiome and the influence it can have on so many things in our body. The microbiome is like a little ecosystem inside our body. It is made up of lots of different types of bacteria which all perform functions. It's been found that some of these bacteria can have positive effects and some have negative. But, it's not just about the bacteria themselves but about what we are feeding these bacteria.

What is the microbiome?

We have around 10 times more bacteria in our guts than cells in our body[28] and it's this bacteria (or microbes) that make up our microbiome. Most of these microbes live in our large intestine (colon) but every part of our body has microbes living in or on it (even our skin). Each of these separate colonies of microbes around our body are known as microbiota.

The majority of these microbes are beneficial and they help us to digest food, such as vegetables, which we wouldn't be able to digest without them, provide energy for our metabolism, make essential vitamins and act as the first line of defence against germs.

Of course, there's also some 'bad' bacteria in our microbiome but the good bacteria in our bodies works to stop the bad ones from growing in too many numbers.

Every day the bacteria in our microbiome looks slightly different as new bacteria enters our body and develops and others leave or die off. And, no two people's microbiomes are the same - not even identical twins.

It is thought we have around 500-1000 different types of bacteria in our bodies - totalling trillions. The role the microbiome plays is wide-reaching and essential to our survival. We are only just beginning to really understand the roles it plays.

Some of its main functions include protecting us from bacteria that cause disease, regulating our immune system and breaking down our food to absorb nutrients. It also produces vitamins (including B12, thiamine, riboflavin and K) and has an influence over whether we are fat or thin, affects our overall health and contributes to our rate of ageing.

An imbalance of the gut microbiota is known as dysbiosis. Dysbiosis may play a role in causing and/or contributing to many diseases, including some beyond the digestive system[29]. These diseases and conditions include irritable bowel syndrome, inflammatory bowel disease, neonatal necrotizing enterocolitis, gastrointestinal (GI) cancers, asthma, allergy, and infectious diseases, Parkinson's Disease, Alzheimer's disease, cancer, obesity and diabetes[30].

Feeding the microbiome

The bugs in our gut respond to the foods we eat. The 'good' bacteria thrive off colourful, plant-based foods, and they love diversity of these types of foods. You may hear people saying they try to 'eat the rainbow'. By this they mean they try to get as many different types and colours of fruit and vegetables into their diet as possible. Similarly highly processed foods and sugar feed the 'bad' bacteria.

"I try to eat as many foods as possible that will feed my microbiome"

Now that I'm able to eat a much wider spectrum of foods I try to eat as many foods as possible that will feed my microbiome. This means avoiding processed or sugar-laden foods, eating lots of fresh fruit, vegetables and protein (such as eggs, meat and fish). I also eat some beans and non-gluten grains (such as rice and quinoa) but not on a daily basis.

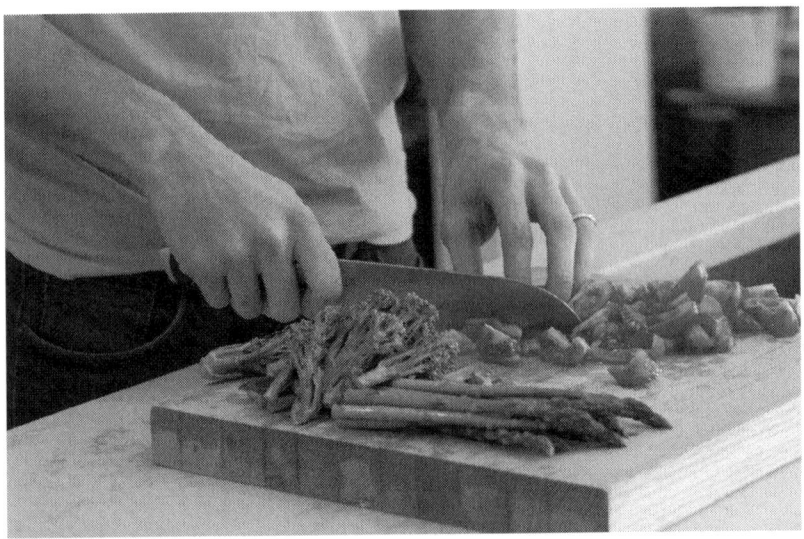

I now eat a range of fruit and vegetables daily. Photograph: Oliver Perrott

I also try to eat probiotic foods to add to my bacterial diversity. Probiotics are live bacteria and yeasts that can be found in some foods and specialist products. I also take a liquid probiotic supplement called Symprove daily. One study into Symprove and ulcerative colitis has been carried out which showed a reduction in faecal calprotectin (an inflammation marker) levels in 76% of participants after 4 weeks[31]. After I started taking this for a few weeks I definitely started to notice a different in my stools and frequency of needing the toilet.

Foods that can help to positively influence the gut microbiome include:

- Fresh vegetables in lots of different colours
- Leafy greens
- Whole fruits (not juice)
- Herbs and spices
- Probiotic foods - some yogurts, sauerkraut, kombucha, kefir
- Good quality fish and meat (wild, grass-fed)
- Nuts and seeds
- Grass-fed butter, extra virgin olive oil, coconut oil
- Red wine and dark chocolate/cocoa (in moderation!)

Treating SIBO

As I learnt more about the microbiome I started to come across small intestinal bacterial overgrowth (SIBO). In SIBO you can end up with excessive bacteria in your small intestine. There are various reasons why it is thought this happens, which include a diet high in sugar and refined carbohydrates (exactly the diet I used to eat) and eating habits. In some people SIBO can cause chronic diarrhoea, weight loss and malabsorption[32]. When I first read about it I was pretty sure that I had it - symptoms include gas, bloating and food intolerances (such as gluten and dairy). Patients with IBD[33], particularly Crohn's disease are at higher risk of developing it[34]. However, SIBO is difficult to diagnose and to treat and I had other things to concentrate on (like getting my IBD under control) and it wasn't for another four years that I finally got around to looking again at SIBO. I spoke to my IBD consultant about my concerns but he said that SIBO testing wasn't available on the NHS where I live. So, I paid to see an experienced nutritionist and functional medicine practitioner (who also helped me with the supplements I talk about later). At this point my IBD was under control but I was still experiencing a lot of gas and bloating. From my symptoms and a stool test she agreed that I was probably suffering from SIBO and started me on a herbal treatment to try to tackle it. After only a few weeks of taking the herbs I noticed a great improvement in my symptoms. I was pleased as the other alternative to treating SIBO is to use antibiotics which wipe out your microbiome (something I didn't want after all the hard work I had been putting into it).

Understanding the digestive system

I also found myself reading more about how the digestive system works. It was something we had touched on in high school science classes but then I'd never given it a second thought after. One thing that really stuck in my mind during my reading was the time it takes for food to pass through our digestive system - 24-72 HOURS, depending on what you've eaten. I'd always associated certain foods (such as salad leaves and tomatoes) with exacerbating my ulcerative colitis symptoms because I'd often need the toilet immediately after eating them. I was under the impression that certain foods would 'go straight through me' - for example if I ate a tomato I'd be on the toilet within 30 minutes. But, if it takes over 24 hours for food to pass through my gut then surely this couldn't be possible, could it? Could this association be in my mind? I wanted to test out this theory so once my bowel had started to heal and I'd reintroduced all other fruit and veg I started eating salad leaves and tomatoes again. It took me a while to get over the anxiety, but I persevered and it didn't take long before I started to be able to eat them without rushing to the toilet straight after. After eating one of these foods I'd make sure I did some deep breathing to try to calm my mind and break the negative association I had made.

It was at this point that I discovered the gastrocolic reflex (also known as the gastrocolic response). This reflex helps to make room for more food in your digestive system. When we eat it stimulates movement in our gastrointestinal tract - which includes contractions in our large intestine to move digested food along. In some people these contractions can then lead to a bowel movement shortly after eating, particularly if your bowel movements are 'loose'. This made sense for me. I would very often need to go to the toilet after eating. Realising this helped me to disassociate salad and tomatoes with needing the toilet.

There were also lots of foods I avoided because I'd see them undigested in my stools. But, when my son started weaning onto solid food I realised that it's quite normal to see undigested bits of food in your poo! We aren't able to digest every single piece of food we eat - especially very high-fibre ones - so the leftovers have to come out of your body somehow! Now that I know it's quite normal to see bits of sweetcorn, carrots, seeds and nuts in poo I'll happily chow down on them.

How digestion works

Mouth: Digestion starts in the mouth before you have even started your meal. When you smell, see or think about tasty food your mouth will often start salivating. When you take your first bite this saliva mixes with the food to help break it down so that your body can absorb it. Chewing the food also aids this process while your tongue moves the food around to get it to your teeth and mix it with the saliva.

Throat: After leaving the mouth the food travels through your throat (also known as the pharynx) towards the esophagus. Esophagus: The esophagus is a muscular tube which connects the throat and the stomach. It is about 25cms long and pushes food down towards your stomach through a series of contractions. It takes 2-3 seconds for the food to move through the esophagus. Just before the point at which the esophagus meets the stomach there is a valve which is designed to stop food from passing back upwards.

Stomach: The stomach is an organ which has strong muscular walls. When the food reaches the stomach it is mixed with acid and powerful enzymes which break down the food. These gastric juices also work to kill bacteria that may be in the food. The stomach has strong wall muscles which help to turn the food into a liquid or paste.

Small intestine (small bowel): After leaving the stomach the food reaches the small intestine. The small intestine is a long tube (more than 6m long and 3.5-5cms wide) which is coiled up in the abdomen. It is made up of three segments - the duodenum, the jejunum and the ileum.

Enzymes from the pancreas and bile from the liver work to continue the process of breaking down the food. Similar to the esophagus, contractions help to move the food through. The job of the duodenum is mostly to continue the process of breaking down the food while the jejunum and ileum are mostly responsible for the absorption of water and nutrients into the bloodstream. Around 90% of digestion and absorption takes place in your small intestine. This is why people with Crohn's disease in their small intestine often suffer from vitamin and mineral deficiencies. Food can spend around 4 hours here. Once the small intestine has absorbed all the nutrients any leftover food moves through to the large intestine (also known as colon).

Large intestine (colon/large bowel): The large intestine is a wide (around 7-10cms) muscular tube that runs between the cecum (the first part of the large intestine) to the rectum (the last part of the large intestine). It is around 1.5m in length. The parts of the large intestine are the cecum (the beginning of the colon) the ascending (right) colon, the transverse (across) colon, the descending (left) colon and the sigmoid colon - which connects to the rectum. Food waste is moved through the large intestine by contractions and as it passes through more water and nutrients are absorbed so that a stool is formed. This stool is then stored in the sigmoid colon until the body empties it into the rectum. It normally takes around 36 hours for a stool to get through the large intestine. A stool is mostly made up of food debris and bacteria. When the descending colon becomes full it empties the contents into the rectum.

Rectum: The rectum connects the colon to the anus. It is around 20cm long and holds the stool until your body is ready to push it out. When a stool or gas reaches the rectum sensors send a message to the brain to let it know that there is something in the rectum. Muscles, known as sphincters, act to hold in the stool until a message is sent from the brain to let the rectum know that the stool can be released. When this happens the muscles relax, releasing the contents.

Anus: The anus is the last part of the digestive tract and the lining of the upper anus works to detect rectal contents and tell your body whether the contents are liquid, gas or solid. The anus is made up of the pelvic floor muscles and two anal sphincters (internal and external muscle rings) work together to stop a stool from coming out. The external sphincter (voluntary) works to keep the stool in until we can get to the toilet while the internal sphincter (involuntary) stops us from going to the bathroom when we are asleep or unaware of the stool. These muscles relax as the stool is expelled.

Why I still don't eat gluten or dairy

I don't have any confirmed allergies to gluten or dairy, yet I've decided to continue not to eat them. This decision was made after doing extensive reading on the subjects, speaking to dieticians and nutritionists and 'experimenting' on myself. If I reintroduce large amounts of dairy and any gluten then I notice a change in my IBD symptoms very quickly. Below is what I've learnt about why this might be...

Gluten

Although I'm not allergic to gluten I do believe I'm gluten sensitive. Whether gluten sensitivity exists is a controversial subject among medics and the media and not something that is yet fully understood. But it's something I strongly believe is real for me. I feel better when I don't eat gluten and have seen the same happen to several of my close family members.

There are a few main reasons why cutting out gluten may make someone feel better:

Sensitive to gluten or one of the other proteins in wheat: If you are sensitive to any of these then your immune system detects those proteins as foreign objects, triggering an immune response, which increase inflammation.

Sensitivity to FODMAPs: FODMAPS - or fermentable oligosaccharides, disaccharides, monosaccharides and polyols - are simple and complex sugars which can be poorly absorbed and cause gastrointestinal symptoms. This happens in people who have dysbiosis or small intestinal bacterial overgrowth (SIBO). Food containing FODMAPs include some fruits, vegetables, milk and wheat.

Zonulin: It has been shown[35], [36] that eating gluten causes your intestinal cells to release more zonulin which is a substance that increases intestinal permeability (leaky gut). Leaky gut is where the gaps between your intestinal cells increase in size. This can then cause larger molecules to get from your intestine (lumen) into the bloodstream. These can be larger pieces of protein or even bacteria. These things are not normally transferred to the bloodstream so your immune system sees them as foreign and mounts an immune response. If your gut is always "leaky" due to eating gluten then you're always going to have this immune response which increases inflammation amongst other things. If we stop eating the gluten and allow the intestinal lining to "heal" then molecules can no longer get into the bloodstream and the immune response can subside.

Through experimentation I know that I'm not sensitive to FODMAPs and I can eat some gluten free products that still contain wheat. However, when I eat gluten I get fatigue and gastrointestinal symptoms - which has led me to believe gluten is a problem for me.

Many people with IBD have tried cutting gluten out of their diets with differing effects. A cross-sectional study[37] in the United States in 2014 found "65.6% of all patients, who attempted a gluten-free diet, described an improvement of their gastrointestinal symptoms and 38.3% reported fewer or less severe IBD flares. In patients currently attempting a gluten free diet, excellent adherence was associated with significant improvement of fatigue".

At the United European Gastroenterology (UEG) Week in 2016 researchers presented findings from a study into a family of proteins in wheat. The researchers said that amylase-trypsin inhibitors (ATIs) - a protein found in wheat, barley and rye - have been shown to trigger an immune response in the gut that can spread to other tissues in the body. They say ATIs have been suggested to exacerbate rheumatoid arthritis, multiple sclerosis (MS), asthma, lupus, and nonalcoholic fatty liver disease, as well as inflammatory bowel disease[38].

Dairy

As with gluten, I have no proven allergy to dairy, however I choose not to eat it as I feel it negatively affects me. But it's something I would like to try experimenting with in the future to see if I can reintroduce some dairy back into my diet.

It is only in recent times that humans have started consuming animal milk and there are many parts of the world (mostly outside of the westernised world) that do not consume animal milk at all. Human adults in areas where animal milk is consumed have evolved to produce the enzyme lactase which allows us to break down the milk sugar lactose. Relatively speaking this is a very recent evolution and some people may not have evolved as much as others in being able to consume it. For example, in China and South East Asia where diary isn't as widely consumed it's thought that up to 90% of people are lactose intolerant[39].

Many people with IBD report their symptoms become worse after consuming dairy products. A study[40] showed that in UC patients the frequency of lactose intolerance was 28.6%, and among Crohn's disease patients 35.3% were considered intolerant. The exact reasons for this are not known.

It is also thought that some people with IBD (particularly those with Crohn's disease affecting the small bowel) have a disruption in production of lactase, particularly when they are having a flare. This disruption can be temporary or permanent. They may also have unbalanced gut bacteria and introducing probiotics could help[41].

Sources of calcium

Dairy is a source of calcium, but it's not the only one. I now ensure I get plenty of the following foods to keep my calcium intake up:

- Seeds (especially poppy, sesame and chia)
- Sardines and canned salmon
- Beans and lentils
- Almonds
- Dark leafy greens (especially collard greens, kale and spinach)
- Edamame beans
- Tofu
- Calcium fortified foods
- Dried figs

It's also important to get enough vitamin D and magnesium to help with calcium intake.

Vitamin D is important to regulate calcium in your body. You get vitamin D from sunshine or you can supplement. Calcium also can't be utilised properly without sufficient magnesium in the body, which is why they are often supplemented together.

If your body doesn't have enough calcium in it then it will start to break down your bones (where lots of calcium is stored) to get what it needs. This is called osteoporosis.

Improving eating habits

It's not just what I eat, but how I eat that I've changed - such as chewing my food more. We chew food to break bigger particles down into smaller ones. This makes it less difficult for your digestive system to process the food. The act of chewing also causes saliva to be produced, which contains digestive enzymes. These enzymes help to break down the food further. The smaller the food particles are as they pass through your small intestine the more nutrients there are available to be absorbed. Digesting food is a very energy consuming process for your body, so by chewing your food more you reduce the amount of energy needed. If pieces of food reach your colon which haven't been chewed properly they can cause gas and bloating. SIBO (as mentioned earlier) can exacerbate this.

When I increased the amount of fibre I was eating I started by making a smoothie out of them. Once I progressed onto eating them I wanted to make it as easy as possible for my digestive system to process the food. So, I started to chew more thoroughly before swallowing. This means I try to chew each mouthful of soft foods 10 times and each mouthful of tougher foods around 30 times.

I've also stopped drinking any liquid while eating. I used to get through a full pint of water at each meal, thinking I was helping the digestive process. However, drinking while eating can actually interfere with digestion. It's thought the liquid can wash the digestive enzymes away before they've had a chance to get to work on the food. The liquid may also have the effect of sweeping food particles through the digestive system before they've been properly broken down into small pieces. Instead I now drink all of my liquids in-between meals.

"It's not just what I eat, but how I eat that I've changed"

I was brought up to always eat dinner at the table, so I've never been a person that eats in front of the TV. However, I had become guilty of eating my lunch at my desk. It's been shown that eating while distracted can lead to increased calorie intake[42]. I wasn't too worried about putting on weight but it did concern me that I might not be getting all the nutrients from my food and causing my body to have to work harder by not chewing well enough because I was distracted. Eating at my desk also meant I was moving around less and getting more pain in my joints and not taking a break from looking at a screen - leading to headaches and increased stress.

Since moving away from my desk at lunchtime I've felt like I have a lot more energy. I've also had less gassy symptoms now that I'm chewing my food more.

The process of being more aware of what, and how, you are eating is known as mindful eating.

Fasting

Fasting is often considered something that people do when they want to lose weight, but it can actually be beneficial for your health, if done correctly. Some IBD patients find themselves doing periods of fasting unintentionally due to severe gastrointestinal symptoms during a flare. I too have done this. For quite a few years I struggled to get my symptoms under control unless I was taking steroids. This often meant I was faecally incontinent. To combat this I used to avoid eating anything around the times I needed to be out of the house (such as at work). I know of other patients who do this too - only eating one meal a day in the evenings because they are worried they will get 'caught short' if they eat when they are away from a toilet. Although I felt weak during this time, probably because I wasn't getting enough nutrients and I was losing a lot of fluid through severe diarrhoea, I did find that my toilet-related symptoms improved when I didn't eat for long periods (such as for 20 hours).

A lot of what we have recently discovered about the positive effects fasting can have on our body is down to Yoshinori Ohsumi. In 2016 he was awarded the Nobel Prize for Medicine in for his work into autophagy - a process that begins when we go without food for around 12 hours. In simple terms autophagy is, essentially, our body's way of housekeeping. During this time the body seeks out old, dead cell matter and breaks them down so they can be reused. Autophagy quickly provides fuel for energy and building blocks for renewal of cellular components[43].

We evolved not to need to eat as regularly as we do now. Back when we were hunter-gatherers and food was much less readily available we would often go for long periods without food. However, now food is so much more readily available we rarely go for several hours without eating. This is often through habit or boredom, rather than necessity.

How hunger works

We need food to survive so our body has developed a way of telling us that we need more food - hunger. There are a number of hormones that are involved in the process of hunger. These hormones help us to make sure we consume the right amount of food and stop us from consuming too much.

When our stomach is empty it releases a hormone called ghrelin. Small amounts of ghrelin are also released by the small intestine, pancreas and brain. Ghrelin is often referred to as the hunger hormone. It stimulates appetite, increases food intake, promotes fat storage and plays a role in insulin release. It is at its highest just before we eat and during fasting and when we eat it is reduced.

Ghrelin has been found to have anti-inflammatory properties

and most animal models with colitis administered with ghrelin were found to have improvements in disease activity and systemic inflammation[44].

Once ghrelin has signalled to our brains that we need food and we have started eating a hormone called leptin is produced by our fat cells. The leptin signals to our brain that we are full. Your small intestine also produces a hormone called Peptide YY (PYY) which suppresses the feeling of hunger.

Eating protein and fibre increases PYY production - thus decreasing the feelings of hunger. However, less PYY is produced when sugary or carbohydrate heavy foods are eaten - increasing the feeling that you need more to eat.

I now do daily 'micro-fasts' in which I try to eat all my food within a 12 hour window (so 7am-7pm) giving my body at least 12 hours' rest every day. I also try to do at least a 24 hour fast every few weeks so that my body gets a longer chance to carry out autophagy. During this time I tend to eat dinner and then don't eat again until the following dinner time. However, before and after this I make sure I eat more nutrients than I usually do (lots of vegetables and good protein). Day-to-day I also listen to my body a lot more. If I'm not hungry I won't eat just because it's lunchtime but I also won't do a longer fast if I wake up and am feeling very hungry and weak.

While reading about fasting I also learnt about the 'migrating motor complex'. This process occurs once your stomach has emptied - about 1-2 hours after eating. The villi (small, finger-like bits of tissue in the small intestine) start to move in a sweeping motion towards the colon. This motion literally sweeps food, enzymes and bacteria along your small intestine towards and into the colon. Essentially your villi are cleaning up your small intestine and clearing out all the debris. This process takes 3-4 hours to complete from when you eat. However, if you eat anything during this time it completely halts the process and must start again. When the body isn't given regular opportunity to do this it's thought the debris contributes to irritable bowel syndrome and SIBO[45].

Before I knew this I used to have some kind of snack around once an hour during the day. This meant the villi weren't being given a chance to do their work during the day and it would only happen once every 24 hours while I was asleep. Now I try to avoid any snacking and leave at least four hours between meals. So, I'm now achieving at least three of these 'sweeps' a day, rather than just the one. I quickly noticed a big difference in reducing heartburn, gassiness and other symptoms when I started spreading out my eating.

One thing I did notice when I first stopped snacking was that at around 11.30am I would suddenly feel quite hungry. After doing some reading I realised this feeling was probably the ileocaecal valve opening to let the food into the colon as the housekeeping cycle finished. Although it actually felt like I was getting hungry, after around 15 minutes the feeling went and I no longer felt any hunger. Before I knew this I would rush for food, which would prevent the process from completing. Now I wait a little while, knowing that eating could actually be counterproductive.

Of course, there are times when I lapse and do have a snack, particularly if I'm craving something or offered something by someone in the office. However, managing to avoid snacking most of the time has had the added bonus of improving my food choices. Although I would make good choices for my meals I tended to make poorer choices (such as sugary foods) as a snack. Now I don't snack I've taken that temptation and choice away.

"The idea that I was potentially adding to the inflammation through the food I was eating scared me"

Controlling blood sugar levels

When making changes to my diet I started doing a lot of reading into sugar and the effect it has on the body. Shortly after my ulcerative colitis diagnosis I became addicted to sweets and chocolate and I found giving them up hard. To do so I needed to know there was a good reason behind why reaching for the Haribo would have a negative effect on my health. Something that seriously caught my attention were various pieces of research which suggest raised blood sugar levels contribute to inflammation in the body. IBD is an inflammatory condition (it's even in the name – inflammatory bowel disease) in which areas of the gut become inflamed. The idea that I was potentially adding to the inflammation through the food I was eating scared me.

A small study of 29 people who drank just one 375ml can of a sugar-sweetened drink over a 3 week period saw an increase in their blood CRP levels (a marker of inflammation)[46]. Another study showed that consuming a 50g dose of fructose caused a spike in inflammation markers (such as CRP mentioned in the previous study) only 30 minutes after consuming it and lasted up to 2 hours after[47].

What is inflammation? ⓘ

Inflammation is your body's response to injury and is an important part of the way our immune system functions. When we cut or hurt ourselves our body sends white blood cells to the area to protect and surround the damaged area. This causes redness and swelling (inflammation) and acts to help protect our body from infection and invading bacteria and viruses. This type of inflammation is known as acute inflammation - it is short-lived. The same reaction occurs when we have a cold or similar illness.

Sustained inflammation is known as chronic inflammation. It is commonplace in autoimmune diseases such as IBD as well as allergies and asthma. When your body has long-term inflammation it can start to damage and attack itself as there are often no invading bacteria or viruses to target. In IBD this can cause damage to your gastrointestinal tract and cause issues in other parts of your body.

Chronic inflammation has been linked to a host of diseases and conditions, including most autoimmune conditions and even depression.

But, it's not just sugar that can drive your blood sugar levels high. Refined flour, refined carbohydrates and grains can do the same. This happens because they are absorbed quickly into the bloodstream which, in turn, causes quick spikes in blood sugar and insulin levels.

Refined carbohydrates and grains include things such as flours and foods made with them (all kinds, although wholemeal flours take longer to absorb so don't spike blood sugar as quickly), white rice, instant rice, pasta, noodles, couscous.

Fruits are also high in sugar - some of the highest being mangoes, cherries, grapes and bananas, however they also contain fibre and vitamins so are a better choice than sweets when you are having a sugar craving.

Artificial sweeteners

Along with giving up sugar I've also stopped eating anything with artificial sweeteners in. I mainly based this decision on a study published in 2014[48] which showed that sweeteners can cause changes to your gut bacteria and the way it metabolises sugar. In mice this made them glucose intolerant (which indicates higher than normal blood sugar levels).

A study published in 2018 found six common artificial sweeteners and 10 sport supplements containing them to be toxic to the digestive gut microbes of mice[49].

Artificial sweeteners include: acesulfame potassium, aspartame, neotame, saccharin, sucralose and stevia/rebaudioside.

Supplements

A few years into my journey, and after I'd made the majority of changes to my diet and lifestyle that I talk about in this book, I started to do some reading about supplements. I'd often see in IBD Facebook groups people asking about the efficacy of various supplements and I'd also started to come across mention of some of them in the reading into nutrition and IBD that I had been doing. Before starting any supplements I always make sure I understand the mechanisms behind what the supplement is supposed to be doing and also look at the published research into it, both specifically for IBD and for general health issues. I also do research into whether a supplement is safe (i.e. can you take too much of it, what side effects might there be). I weigh all of these up before making a decision as to whether to take it or not. In making my decisions about supplements I have also enlisted the help of an experienced, well-qualified nutritionist and functional medicine practitioner and also spoken with my IBD consultant about what I am doing.

With supplements it can be difficult to tell if something is having an effect as the changes may be slow and gradual. This is especially the case if you had a severe deficiency when you started taking it and time is needed to build up your reserves to an optimal level. It's also difficult to know what the correct dose to take is as there is very little 'official' advice on what a therapeutic dose should be. This is where the nutritionist was particularly helpful in helping me find the correct dose and making sure I was choosing the right supplements for me, and wasn't wasting money on an expensive product. It was also helpful to get their advice on which brands of supplement to buy. There are so many companies these days capitalising on the boom in the supplement industry and there is a huge range in the quality of the products they supply. I wanted to ensure the products I was using were the highest quality I could find.

When I started taking these supplements my IBD and general health was already in a place that I was happy with. I was in symptomatic remission (I hadn't yet had a colonoscopy to confirm clinical remission) and feeling fairly good day-to-day. However, since taking these supplements I've noticed an even further improvement in how I feel. I now have fully formed stools (something I haven't had for over ten years) and I wake up every day fully energised. However, this may be a coincidence, rather than a result of taking the supplements.

For information only I've listed below the supplements I take and the research and reasons behind why I take them.

Vitamin D

Vitamin D helps to regulate the amount of calcium and phosphate in the body and is essential for healthy bones. It also plays a role in reducing inflammation and is important for good general health and growth. Vitamin D is produced in our body when our skin is exposed to sunlight. There are studies which have shown a link between people with inflammatory bowel disease (IBD) having lower levels of vitamin D than the general population[50]. It is one of the most common vitamin deficiencies seen in people with Crohn's disease. A five-year study published in 2016 found that low levels of vitamin D in people with IBD is associated with high disease severity[51]. In the UK Public Health England recommends people consider supplementing with vitamin D during the winter months when we aren't exposed to sunlight[52]. Because of this, and the research which indicates higher disease severity in people with low levels of vitamin D, I started supplementing daily with a vitamin D spray. I take my dose in the morning when we should usually be getting exposure to sunlight.

Magnesium

Magnesium is important in more than 300 chemical reactions to keep the body working. These include growth and maintenance of bones, function of nerves, muscles and many other parts of the body. In the stomach magnesium helps to neutralise stomach acid and moves stools through the intestine. Magnesium deficiency is not uncommon among the general population (around two-thirds of the western world are not thought to be reaching daily allowances of magnesium[53]) and magnesium deficiency can be common among people with inflammatory bowel disease (IBD)[54]. I've used magnesium transdermally (absorption through the skin) via baths and magnesium sprays for around four years. I started this as a way to relax my muscles and aid with sleep. It wasn't until I was in remission that I started taking it orally, due to the effect it can have on your digestive system (increased bowel movements). Following a blood test which showed I was at the lower end of the range for magnesium I started supplementing orally. It may also benefit sleep, as mentioned earlier in this book.

Turmeric

Studies have shown that curcumin (found in the root of turmeric) is a 'promising and safe therapy for maintaining remission in patients with quiescent UC as well as for improving symptoms in patients with proctitis and CD (Crohn's disease)'[55]. It is also thought to inhibit the inflammatory process[56] . I now take curcumin daily in tablet form. I also try to use turmeric in cooking whenever possible, though you need quite a lot of turmeric each day to gain benefits from it, which is why I also take the tablets. When taking turmeric you also need to have it with black pepper or it won't be absorbed fully into your body.

L-glutamine

L-glutamine is an amino acid, although not considered to be an essential amino acid. It helps essential processes in the body, particularly at times of stress.

It is important for providing nitrogen and carbon to many different cells. Nitrogen is needed after surgery or injury to repair the wounds and keep vital organs functioning. It is made in muscles and if more L-glutamine is used than the body can make then muscle wasting can occur. Studies have shown that oral glutamine supplementation supports gastrointestinal mucosal growth and is considered the most important nutrient for healing of 'leaky gut syndrome'[57]. Leaky gut is a condition in which the small intestine membrane has become porous (or leaky) allowing toxins, microbes, undigested food particles and antibodies to pass through and travel around your body in your bloodstream. L-glutamine has also been found to lessen the severity of diarrhoea by enhancing water and salt intake[58].

Methylsulfonylmethane (MSM)

MSM is an organic sulphur which helps build healthy bones and joints. There have been various studies which show MSM has a huge range of benefits including improved skin health, exercise recovery, joint support and allergy/immunity support[59]. I started taking MSM as I was suffering from muscle pains and poor muscle recovery following exercise. Studies show that MSM can reduce muscle damage in exercise[60] and that it helps exercise recovery[61]. Since taking it I have noticed a reduction in the pain I have been getting, however as I also do a lot of other things to help with the pain (such as stretching and massaging) I can't be sure it's the MSM that has had a positive effect.

Colostrum

Colostrum is the first milk created by a mother when a baby is born. It contains antibodies and immune factors that the mother passes to the baby. Colostrum supplements are taken from the milk of grass-fed cows, known as bovine colostrum. Bovine colostrum contains many of the same nutrients that are found in human colostrum.

It is a rich source of nutrients, antibodies and growth factors and a small study has shown that it's use (albeit as an enema) could have benefits for distal (left-sided) colitis[62].

An animal study[63] and a very small human study[64] have shown there are benefits for UC in taking colostrum, however more research is needed.

Fibre

I've already mentioned earlier that I've now increased my fibre intake to help support my microbiome. But, there have also been some studies which show fibre can help with IBD[65], with one study showing that people with Crohn's disease who did not avoid high fibre foods were 40% less likely to have a disease flare than those who avoided high fibre foods[66]. Another study[67] concluded that "certain types of dietary fibre in conjunction with medication would appear appropriate in helping to control disease symptoms".

Fibre is a natural substance that primarily comes from

the cell walls of plants. The substance, cellulose, is very similar to sugar but humans don't have the enzyme to break it down. It is impossible for a human to digest. However, some bacteria in our guts are able to break it down (ferment) as their food or "prebiotic" and create useful byproducts for us such as the short chain fatty acid "butyrate", which is associated with lower colorectal cancer risk[68]. Different prebiotics feed different microbes. If our aim is to have a diverse, healthy microbiota then eating lots of different kinds of fibres/prebiotics will help feed our microbiota.

High fibre diets have also been found to increase the number of T cells (Tregs) than a low fibre diet[69]. It's thought this happens because butyrate promotes the formation of Tregs. Tregs are important because they help suppress inflammatory responses.

Fibre is also important for keeping our digestive system healthy and prevents constipation. Fibre can bulk up stools, make stools softer and make it easier for them to move through the colon. Because it helps to move waste out of our digestive system it means the amount of time waste products are in contact with the bowel is reduced. This is thought to be one of the reasons why eating fibre reduces risk of bowel cancer.

Increase water and electrolyte intake

Water is essential to keep us alive. Our bodies are made up of around 60% water. Nearly all the major systems in our body depend on water to function - it helps regulate our temperature, keeps our eyes, nose and mouth moist, lubricates joints, helps flush out waste products through the liver and kidneys and carries nutrients and oxygen to cells. It's pretty important stuff. But throughout the day we lose water through sweating, breathing and digestion so we need to keep topping up our water levels.

I always knew that it was important for me to be drinking water regularly, especially when I was in a flare and losing even more water through diarrhoea. Despite this I'd always still feel thirsty and get headaches which felt like I was de-hydrated. It wasn't until I started adding a pinch of sea salt to some of the water I was drinking that these symptoms started to go away.

The salt adds trace minerals which help to hold more water in my body, quenching my thirst for longer. I always make sure I use sea or rock salt rather than table salt as it isn't processed which removes these beneficial minerals. Now, whenever I have a thirst that I can't quench I add a little salt to my water for a while and it soon abates.

Steps to getting a more balanced diet with IBD

Getting to the point where I can now eat pretty much all forms of fruit, vegetables, nuts and seeds has taken years. It's helped by the fact that I'm now in remission, but even during my last flare (July 2017) I was still able to eat many of the foods I previously avoided. When I first started try-ing to eat a more nutrient dense diet I used some different techniques to slowly ease my gut into it. These included:

Blending

I would peel and blend a host of fruit and vegetables with some water to make a smoothie. As I became more confident with this I started adding some of the peel to the mix until I wasn't peeling anything at all.

Stewing

I would eat stewed fruits such as apples, pears, rhubarb, berries etc. Again, I started without any peel and slowly added this in.

Roasting

I still eat a lot of roasted vegetables. On a Sunday I often cook a huge tray of sweet potatoes, parsnips, carrots, beetroot and butternut squash in olive or coconut oil. These are then kept in the fridge and throughout the week I use them as a quick and nutritious accompaniment to meat or fish. Roasting the vegetables helps to soften them, thus aiding the digestion process.

Protein powders

I would use a protein powder in my smoothie to help make sure I was getting enough protein to support my body. I tended to use Puriton's plant-based protein powders that are dairy free and low in sugar/sweeteners.

Nut butters

I've never had too many problems with eating nuts as long as I chew them well, but often if I was in a flare I would use nut butter as an alternative way to get the good fats contained in nuts. I also often add it to stir frys with some tamari (gluten free soy sauce) to add a nutty taste.

Don't buy junk

I have literally no willpower when it comes to some foods (generally chocolate!) so I have a rule that I don't keep any processed or sugar-laden foods in the house. If they aren't there I can't eat them!

Healthy snacks

When I used to snack I made sure I had some healthy options readily available so I wasn't tempted to buy a bar of chocolate or cake. These snacks included trail mix, olives, nuts, boiled eggs, fruit and seeds.

Learn to read labels

I found part of the battle was understanding the labels on foods. They often include so many ingredients I've never even heard of. I ended up learning what all the different types of gluten containing grains were, the many different names for sugar and sweeteners and the different types of fats. Now, though, I try to buy as much fresh food as possible so I don't have to worry about labels.

When I first started eating a more nutrient dense diet I became a bit obsessed by it. It consumed a lot of my thoughts and I would beat myself up if I ate something that wasn't 'good for me'. It became a real chore and I started losing the enjoyment out of food. This stress wasn't good for me (and especially for my UC) so I had to learn to relax a bit about it. I now work on a 90% rule - I aim to follow my diet for around 90% of the time. This allows me to have some treats but also means I don't stray too far. If I am going to have a treat then it's often a small bar of dark chocolate (the darker the better) or the occasional glass of red wine. I do look forward to these treats, but I've also found that my taste buds have changed and I no longer crave sugary snacks in the way I used to. Of course, I'm human - and I have times when I have a complete blow out (but I never eat gluten or dairy) - though I nearly always regret it as my health ultimately suffers.

My diet and nutrition takeaways

Here's a summary of the changes I've made to my diet and nutrition:

- Increased vegetable and fibre intake. I started with a daily smoothie
- Cut out dairy and gluten
- Reduce processed foods

- Reduce sugar and sweeteners

- Reduce refined carbs and grains

- Educated myself about the digestive system

- Fed my gut microbiome

- Take a probiotic

- Treated my small intestinal bacterial overgrowth (SIBO)

- Eat more healthy fats

- Increase fibre slowly into my diet

- Daily 'micro fasts' and regular longer fasts

- Eat nutrient dense, not a calorie dense, diet

- Chew food more thoroughly

- No eating at desk (or in front of TV)

- Take supplements (vitamin D, magnesium, turmeric, L-glutamine, MSM and colostrum)

Movement and exercise

Exercise has always played a big part in my life. At school I played football, and I have always loved mountain biking and trials riding (a type of biking). When I first became seriously ill with my ulcerative colitis I was told I probably wouldn't be able to exercise in the way I had previously been doing. This was such a huge blow to me. I used exercise as a way of relieving stress and have always felt compelled to do it to keep well. So, I decided I wasn't going to let my UC stop me and continued playing football anyway. However, I certainly noticed some differences. I became tired more easily and my recovery period after exercise was a lot longer than my peers. I also started getting muscle pains and cramps that I hadn't previously experienced. I wasn't sure how much of this was due to the ulcerative colitis itself and how much of this may be a side effect of the medications I was taking. But, for many years I just accepted that this was my new normal and would exercise through the pain or come home and sleep for a few hours after playing a football match.

"When I first became seriously ill with my ulcerative colitis I was told I probably wouldn't be able to exercise in the way I had previously been doing"

However, after starting to adjust my diet (see diet and nutrition section) and feeling a bit better I noticed my capacity to exercise also improved. I started doing more athletics-based exercise and became more interested in stretching to aid with flexibility, warming up and cooling down. The more reading I did the more I discovered exercises that helped with the muscle pains I was experiencing. My main problems were in my legs and arms - mostly tightness and cramping. I noticed that when I wasn't able to exercise or stretch these pains would be a lot worse. My sleep would also be worse and I'd feel generally restless.

Exercise to improve IBD symptoms

Very little research has been carried out into IBD and exercise. However, more studies are now starting to take place.

A review article on the role of physical exercise in IBD concluded: 'Preliminary studies demonstrate that moderate exercise has no negative health effects and may diminish some symptoms of IBD....exercise is recommended also because it could counteract some IBD specific complications by improving immunological response, psychological health, nutritional status, bone mineral density and reversing the decrease of muscle mass and strength'[70].

And many people with IBD that I've spoken to do report that doing exercise gives them more energy, helps them psychologically, reduces muscle and joint pain, and increases muscle and bone strength.

A study has also shown that exercise reduces the risk rate for colon cancer by as much as 50%[71] - and people with IBD in the colon are at a greater risk of developing colon cancer[72]. And, another study found that as little as 20 minutes of exercise can have an anti-inflammatory effect on the body[73].

So, it seems that exercise could play a positive role in IBD. But, the intensity of any exercise you do may be important. Very intense or extreme exercise can cause diarrhoea[74], cramps and bloating in anyone (often found to happen in long-distance runners) and can speed up the transit of stools through the colon - not something you want to happen if you are already experiencing diarrhoea.

I certainly fall into the category of finding positive effects from exercising. The main exercise I do is sprint training. This can be very intensive but only for very short periods (under a minute at a time) which means it doesn't place too much stress on my body and exacerbate my IBD. This type of training is call HIIT (high-intensity interval training). I enjoy these short bursts of activity much more than I've ever enjoyed longer exercise sessions.

I do my HIIT through a short distance sprint followed by a slow walk for recovery, followed by another short sprint etc. But running isn't the only way you can do HIIT. Any form of intense exercise for a short period (such as cycling, boxing, or using cardio machines at the gym) followed by what's known as 'active recovery' (exercising at a slower pace) is HIIT. During these intense periods I find that the only thing I am able to concentrate on is completing the activity I'm doing it's almost like a form of meditation because everything else is gone from my brain. If I go for a longer, slower run I find that I end up thinking about things that have happened during the day or things that I need to get done. The intense bursts also seem to stretch out my body better than a slower bout of exercise would. HIIT also has the added bonus that I can fit a few quick 'rounds' into a spare 10 minutes - whereas I wouldn't get much benefit from a 10 minute jog.

HIIT has been subject of many studies in recent years and, among other things, has shown to modulate blood sugar spikes following a meal[75], improve vascular function[76], improve age related muscle decline[77] and have anti-inflammatory effects[78]. A few pieces of research are also currently taking place specifically into the area of HIIT and IBD... watch this space!

A recent piece of research also interestingly showed that exercise can alter the microbiome[79] that we learnt about in the section on diet and nutrition.

Exercise and movements for pain management

The other type of exercise/movement I do apart from HIIT is to help with muscle pains and cramps. As often as I can I do a series of stretches to relieve pain in my legs, hips and arms. For this I often use resistance bands, pressure point balls and foam rollers to work on areas that are particularly tight or painful. The balls and foam rollers work in a similar way to someone massaging your muscles. I find that by doing stretching and rolling I get pain relief and increased movement in these areas. I definitely notice if I don't do my stretches for a few days. I also use magnesium oil on painful muscles (particularly my legs) to help relax them before I go to bed.

Going barefoot

There's a growing number of people who are going 'barefoot'. The idea is that we should let our feet be free more frequently, rather than keeping them cooped up in too-tight, ill-fitting shoes. There's even a few companies who make 'barefoot' shoes which are designed to feel like you aren't wearing anything on your feet.

When I first starting started hearing about this movement I was very skeptical. I really wasn't convinced that walking around barefoot could have a positive impact on my health. However, one day, during a lunch break, I found myself at

my local beach. It was quite warm and the sea looked invit-
ing. I decided to take my shoes off and walk across the pebbles down to the water. Walking on the stones was incredibly painful but eventually I made it down to the sea. My feet
were burning and aching, but it felt pretty good. Shortly
after this I was on the beach with my toddler son and I saw
that he practically ran across the same stones I had struggled across without giving them a second thought. It got me
thinking that at some point from when I was young to now
my feet had stopped being able to handle walking on the
pebbles. Could it be that years of wearing shoes had something to do with it?

I now walk around barefoot (or just in my socks) whenever
possible and I have to say that my feet do feel better for it.
I haven't gone as far as walking around town in bare feet
but I am now the proud owner of four (or is it five?) pairs of
'barefoot' shoes from a company called Vivobarefoot (and
they are the most comfortable things I've ever worn, I'd
highly recommend them!).

Since that experience on the beach I've done a bit of
research into why going barefoot could be better for our
health, and it does make sense. From an evolutionary point
of view our feet were made to be free. Also having your feet
closer to the ground (or touching it) gives greater sensory
feedback to your brain meaning you are less likely to move
clumsily. For your feet to function properly and provide
your body support in the way they were designed the toes
need to be able to spread out - if they are crammed into
tight shoes then this can't happen and the natural functions of your feet can become impaired. Many shoes are also

quite rigid which prevents our feet from carrying out their natural motion.

Why not try taking your shoes off more often? I promise you won't regret it!

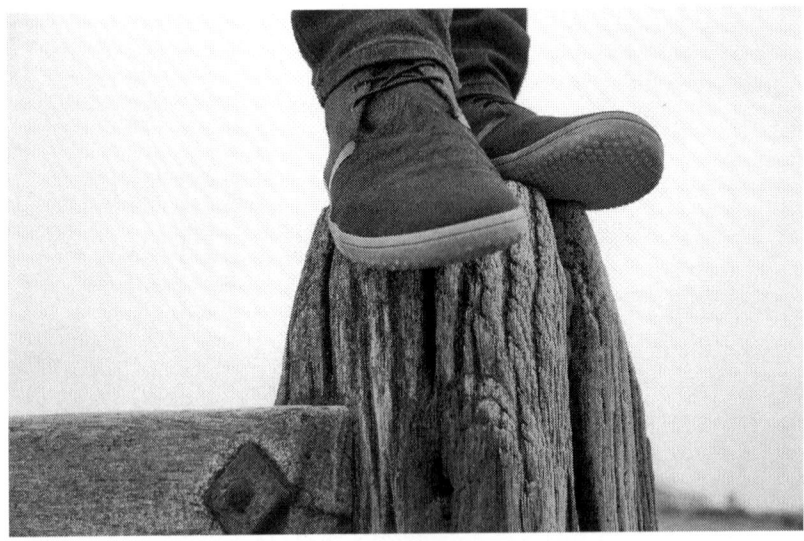

I now wear barefoot shoes most of the time. Photograph: Oliver Perrott

How I fit movement into my life

One of the hardest things I find about keeping active is fitting it into my already busy life. Like many people, when I don't have much time it's exercise that gives way for other things. After years of being an exercise yo-yoer, where I would get into a good routine and then something would happen and I'd get out of the habit I've learnt to build movement into my everyday life, rather than just having specific times that I exercise. As I've previously mentioned

I now have a standing desk at work. This means I naturally move about more and don't spend hours on end being inactive sitting at a desk. Even the act of just standing still is a workout for your body. Each hour at work I make sure I take a short break. During this time I will go for a short walk, do a few stretches, go up and down the stairs a few times - anything to make sure I'm moving my body. I've also started cycling to a client's office I regularly work in and have joined a gym near their office which I'll go to in my lunch break a couple of times a week for half an hour and do a quick few weights or rounds of HIIT.

"Like many people when I don't have much time it's exercise that gives way for other things"

I've also recently got a tracker watch which counts how many steps I'm doing throughout the day. I'm quite a competitive person so each day I try to do more steps than the previous day - and at a minimum I always try to do 10,000. In the evenings I'll do my stretching/muscle rolling while watching TV or talking to my wife about the day, or if it's a nice evening I'll head out on my trials or mountain bike. The main thing I try to do is just always keep moving. I avoid having long periods of being static. But, I also always try to listen to my body. Sometimes my body just doesn't feel capable of doing all of these and I know it's important that I listen to it. Doing too much can be just as detrimental to health as doing too little. So, on days when I'm just not feeling it I'll stick to some gentle stretching and walking.

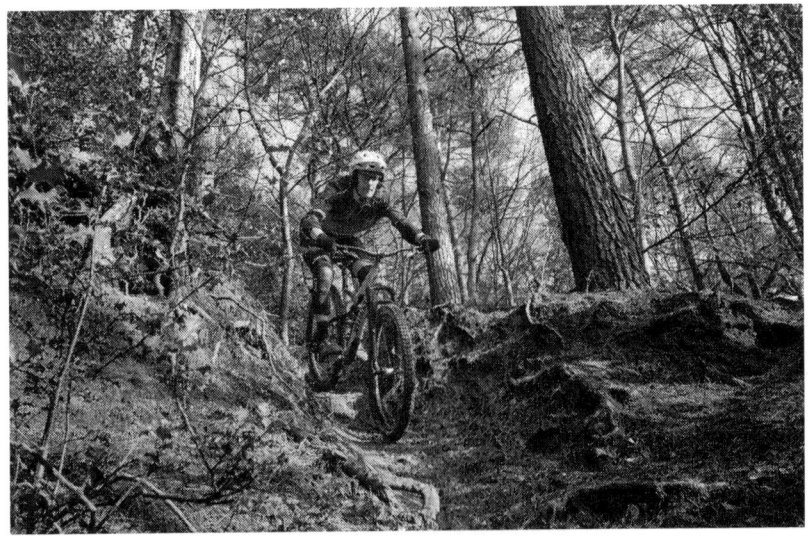

Mountain biking helps my body feel better and acts as a stress reliever.
Photograph: Oliver Perrott

My movement takeaways

Here's a summary of changes I've made to my exercise and movement:

- Use stretching to help with pain
- Use HIIT as preferred exercise (sprint running)
- Use trigger point balls and foam rollers on tight muscles
- Spray magnesium oil on painful muscles
- Go barefoot whenever possible

- Use a standing desk at work

- Move as often as possible

- Go to gym to do short lunchtime sessions

- Cycle/walk to work

- Try to get as many steps each day as possible

- Don't spend long periods being inactive

- Listen to body - doing too much can be as bad as not doing enough

Environment

It's not known exactly what causes IBD but many believe the environment around us plays a part in its development. A study published in 2016 concludes that 'environment plays a major role in the development and activity of IBD'[80] and that more clinical studies into this area are needed. In the UK a study called PREdiCCT is currently taking place to 'increase understanding of how environmental factors, diet, and the gut microorganisms influence inflammatory bowel disease flare and recovery'[81].

But, it's not just IBD that our environment might be having an impact on. Our general health could be suffering too. In 2009 two researchers on the subject wrote: "Environmental degradation poses a significant threat to human health worldwide"[82].

An important step on my journey to improving my health was to look at my environment and consider what I could do to change it to the advantage of my health and well-being.

A lot of the changes I've made are very small but when I add all these changes up I feel (unscientifically!) that they make a big different to my general health.

"Environment plays a major role in the development and activity of IBD"

What environmental factors may have an impact on health?

In the context of health our environment means the air we breathe, what we eat and drink, the stress we face, toxins and chemicals we come into contact with. These can come into your body through breathing, ingesting or contact with your skin. From an evolutionary point of view we would have come into contact with toxins regularly (such as poisonous plants) and our bodies, especially our organs, developed ways of coping with these toxins. However, the toxins we are now facing are significantly different. Instead of the poisons from plants we are now faced with various chemicals in the products we use and pollutants in the air. Humans are very resilient and our bodies have learnt to eliminate a lot of these toxins. However, doing so places a great amount of stress on our bodies. And, as explored earlier in this book, stress is not good for our health.

The impact all of these environmental things are having on

me is something that I've only relatively recently started exploring. I found I was making progress in my health
without making too many changes to my environment,
however it's now an area I've turned my attention too as
the quest for optimal health has become a little addictive
(and, some would say, obsessive!).

Below I've outlined what changes I've made to my environment so far, but I know there's still much more I can do in
this area. But, right now I'm relatively happy with what I
am doing.

Changes I've made to my environment

Water

I've been drinking only filtered water for around 4
years now. Although I actually quite liked the taste of
tap water I started drinking filtered water based on a
recommendation from someone else with IBD. After
doing it for a few weeks I found my bowels seemed
more settled when I was drinking filtered water.

Water quality varies from location to location depending on the company providing the water and the
area's laws. I've read various scare-mongering articles
online about the effect chemicals which could be in our
drinking water may have on health (including chlorine
to clean it, heavy metals from the pipes it travels in,
flouride to keep our teeth healthy). However, the evidence for this isn't clear cut. Both asthma and derma-
titis have been associated with exposure to chlorine[83].

But, my main concern was as to whether the chemicals in the water could be having a negative effect on my gut bacteria. I wondered whether the chlorine, so good at killing germs, could be killing some of the bacteria in my microbiome. I found that the research into whether this is the case is currently limited, though a lot of people seem to have made an assumption that this is an entirely possible outcome. I decided drinking filtered water was not going to do me any harm so I started doing it.

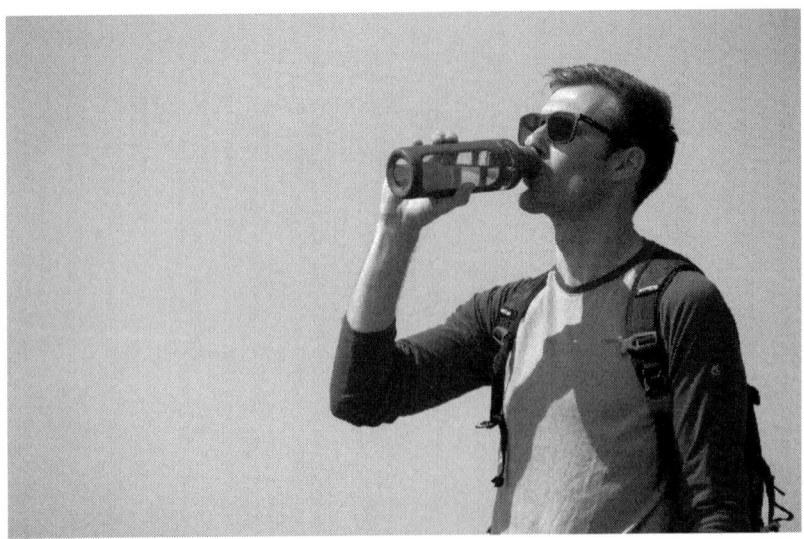

I carry filtered water, in a glass bottle, everywhere with me

I now don't touch tap water unless I really have to. I use filtered water for drinking, cooking and even to wash and cook fruit and vegetables. At home I have installed a Brita filtered water tap. At some point I'd like to upgrade this to a reverse osmosis filtration system.

However, this is a much larger and more expensive option! At my office I have a water filter jug and I also carry a reusable bottle with filtered water in everywhere I go.

Air

The air we breathe can be full of pollutants and toxins, both inside and outside our homes. Things such as fumes from cars and factories, aerosol sprays, cleaning products, mold and damp in our homes and air fresheners can all affect our health via the air we are breathing. It's a fact of our modern lives that we are going to breathe in these things - there's no escape. But, research shows that breathing polluted air can put you at higher risk of various respiratory illnesses[84].

England's Chief Medical Officer Sally Davies wrote in her 2017 Annual Report[85] that 'there are no aspects of our life that do not have the potential to be impacted by pollution' and that she is 'surprised by how little we know about many of the common pollutants that surround us each day'. She also wrote: 'It is clear: the evidence base around the health harms caused by many individual pollutants is not strong. Many of the professionals I spoke to when researching this report, however, raised real concerns about pollutants; and we must remember that the absence of evidence is not evidence of absence'.

What are VOCs? ⓘ

Volatile Organic Compounds, or VOCs, are gases emitted from some solids or liquids. These gases include a variety of organic chemicals and some of them are believed to cause short or long-term health issues.

Household products such as paint, solvents, aerosol sprays, disinfectants, air fresheners, hobby supplies and dry-cleaned clothing all include them. They are also found in building materials and furnishings, photocopiers, printers, correction fluids, glues, adhesives and permanent markers. VOCs may also be released into the air during the manufacture process of some products.

According to the United States Environmental Protection Agency[86] health effects of VOCs may include:

- Eye, nose and throat irritation
- Headaches, loss of coordination and nausea
- Damage to liver, kidney and central nervous system
- Some organics can cause cancer in animals, some are suspected or known to cause cancer in humans.

In a bid to take control of some of the air that I'm breathing I've bought several portable air filters for my house and office. I also never use air fresheners or scented candles (except for those scented by essential oils) as these are packed full of chemicals. And, when I'm doing DIY, such as painting, sanding, drilling etc, I always wear a face mask to protect my lungs.

Damp and mould

Mould and damp are caused by excessive moisture in a building. All buildings will contain some level of moisture, but in some properties this can build up, causing areas of damp to form. If left untreated this can lead to mould build up. You may notice condensation on windows - tell-tale sign that there is moisture in your home or other buildings.

Many of us spend a lot of time inside, whether it's at home or at work, and if there is damp and/or mould present it could be causing us ill-effects. A review by the World Health Organisation (WHO) states "increased prevalences of respiratory symptoms, allergies and asthma as well as perturbation of the immunological system" are "associated with building moisture and biological agents"[87], such as mould.

Some people are thought to be more sensitive to the effects of mould than others. WHO says that "babies and children, elderly people, those with existing skin problems, such as eczema, or respiratory problems, such as allergies and asthma, and anyone who is immunocompromised"[88], such as those on certain medications used in IBD to suppress the immune system, are among those that are more sensitive.

If you have damp or mould in your home it's important that you identify the source and deal with it, otherwise it will continue to return. To help reduce some of the moisture in the air you should ventilate the property regularly (by opening windows and doors) and you can use dehumidifiers or air filters to help get rid of moisture and toxins in the air.

Chemicals

Our bodies are exposed to so many chemicals every day. Each time we wash our hands, hair or body we are bombarded with chemicals from the various personal and beauty products we are using, including those made for children. As these chemicals enter our body (usually via our skin) they need to be broken down or eliminated. Some of these chemicals in our beauty products are inocuos but there are others, such as parabens, synthetic colours, fragrances, phthalates, triclosan, sodium lauryl sulfate (SLS), formaldehyde, toluene and propylene glycol, which have had concerns raised about them in relation to the effects they have on our health. There's very little, if any, regulation surrounding what goes into the products we use on our bodies, which means companies are able to use whatever they like.

Some of these chemicals have become known as endocrine disrupting chemicals (EDCs) and according to the World Health Organisation (WHO) have been 'suspected to be associated with altered reproductive function in males and females; increased incidence of breast cancer, abnormal growth patterns and neurodevelopmental delays in children, as well as changes in immune function'[89].

After learning that I could be putting my body under strain just by using everyday things such as hand sanitiser, shampoo, sunscreen and lip balm I decided to try to make a conscious effort to reduce the number of chemicals I was exposing my body to. To do this I needed to find alternatives, as I wasn't just going to stop washing myself! So I started using organic castile soap (which I scent with essential oils) as hand and body wash and a recipe of beeswax and coconut oil as lip balm. I also started using a natural salt deodorant. I was skeptical about using these products at first as I wasn't sure how effective they would be, but I haven't had any complaints from people around me about their effectiveness so far!

I've also started using an app called Think Dirty which helps to identify some of the personal products which are the worst offenders in terms of potentially harmful chemical usage. Through this I've switched a few of the products we use in our house to different brands.

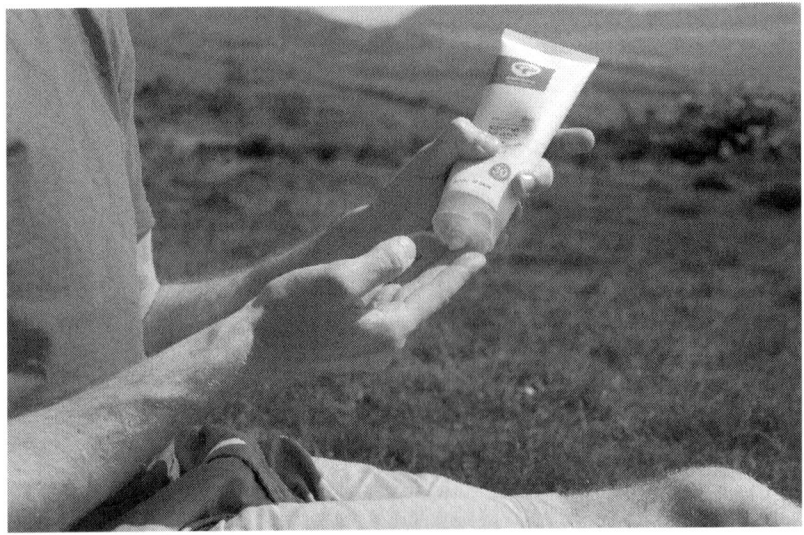

Switching to a non-toxic sunscreen is one of the product changes I've made

Food

I also worry about the toxins in our food. Vegetables and fruit are often sprayed with pesticides to stop them getting attacked by insects as they are growing. It isn't possible for all of these toxins to be washed off so I have started buying as many organic fruit and vegetables as I can. I am a meat eater and I also buy organic meat wherever possible. Many animals are given antibiotics and other medications, which I worry can end up in our bodies. Although the evidence around whether organic food is actually better for us or not isn't clear cut I've decided that I'd prefer not to take any risks with it. I'm now also in a position where I'm able to spend a bit more money on the food I'm eating, something which wasn't the case a few years ago.

Heavy metals

I have bad teeth. I've always had bad teeth but more so since I was diagnosed with IBD. I think a combination of chronic inflammation in my body and years of taking steroids (which have an effect on how your body metabolises calcium and vitamin D) have taken their toll on my mouth. As a result I have a lot of fillings. Many of these used to be mercury-based (amalgam).

I'd read that 'The effects of mercury on the gastrointestinal system typically present as abdominal pain, indigestion, inflammatory bowel disease, ulcers and bloody diarrhea'[90]. The World Health Organisation (WHO) also states that mercury is toxic to human health[91] and the various different forms of mercury can have effects on the nervous, digestive and immune systems and on lungs, kidneys, skin and eyes. This obviously concerned me and got me thinking about the fact that I had mercury permanently in my mouth. I have now been slowly having my mercury fillings replaced with non-toxic fillings.

Filtering my water (as discussed earlier in this book) has the added bonus of reducing any heavy metals being added to my body - such as mercury - that may be found in drinking water.

My environment takeaways

Here's a summary of the things I've done to support better environment:

- Filter drinking water
- Use air filters around the home
- Wear face mask when doing DIY
- Use Think Dirty app and make personal product swaps
- Make own soaps and lip balm
- Eat organic where possible
- Remove mercury fillings

Products I love

Here are lists of the products I have mentioned in this book or other products I like using/have used. I've also included a list of books I've found helpful on my journey.

Please note, all of the links are affiliate links. This means if you buy from the company I may receive a commission. You will pay the same price as you normally would and any money earned will be used to support IBDrelief's work.

Probiotics

I take Symprove everyday and feel it has contributed towards helping me to maintain remission and reduce some of the abdominal symptoms I previously had.

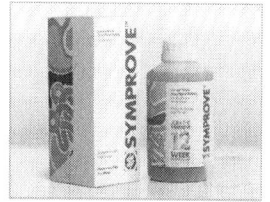

Symprove
https://ibdrelief.com/o/symprove

Supplements

Below are the supplements I use:

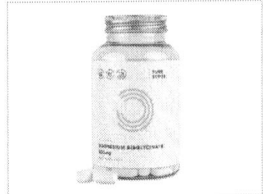

Magnesium glycinate tablets
BULK POWDERS
https://ibdrelief.com/o/mg-tablets

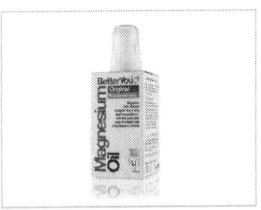

Transdermal magnesium spray
BetterYou
https://ibdrelief.com/o/mg-spray

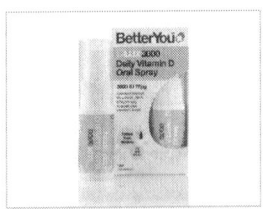

Vitamin D
BetterYou
https://ibdrelief.com/o/vit-d

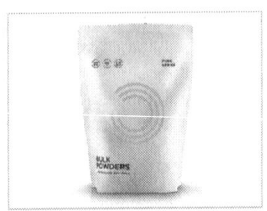

Glutamine
BULK POWDERS
https://ibdrelief.com/o/glutamine

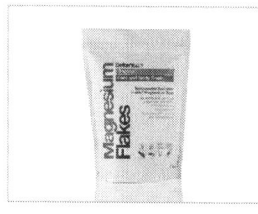

Magnesium flakes
BetterYou
https://ibdrelief.com/o/mg-flakes

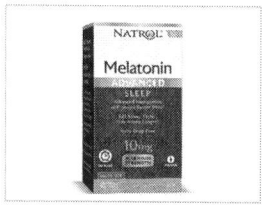

Melatonin
Natrol
https://ibdrelief.com/o/melatonin

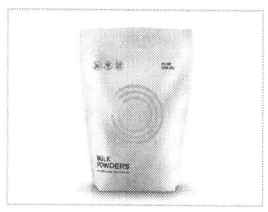

Methylsulfonylmethane (MSM)
BULK POWDERS
https://ibdrelief.com/o/msm

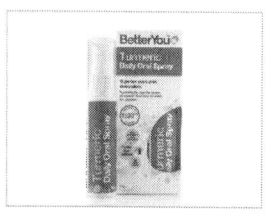

Turmeric
BetterYou
https://ibdrelief.com/o/tumeric

I take the bovine colostrum from Moss Nutrition below, but BULK POWDERS also do one which is more readily available and cheaper (but I haven't personally tried it).

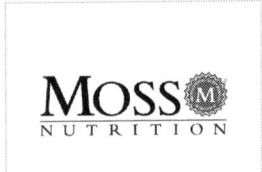

Colostrum
Moss Nutrition
https://ibdrelief.com/o/colostrum

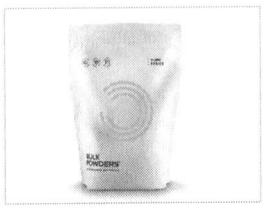

Colostrum
BULK POWDERS
https://ibdrelief.com/o/colostrum-bp

Protein powder

When I'm making smoothies I put a scoop or two of this protein powder in with my fruit and veg if I'm feeling particularly hungry or in a flare.

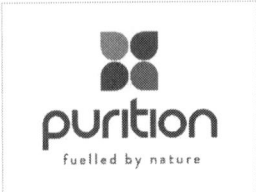

Puriton
https://ibdrelief.com/o/protein

Smoothie making

I don't make so many smoothies now that I'm able to eat fruit and veg in their natural state, but for a long time my Nutri Ninja would get a daily workout (sometimes even twice a day).

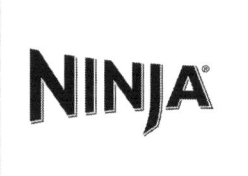

Nutri Ninja
https://ibdrelief.com/o/nutrininja

Water filter

At home we have a Brita filter tap in our kitchen so that filtered water is always available. I would love to get a reverse osmosis filter, though cost and available space has stopped me so far! At my office I have a refillable water filter jug and I've also used their water filter bottle.

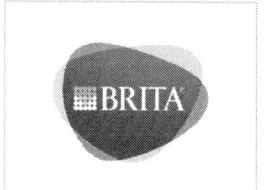

Brita
https://ibdrelief.com/o/brita

Mattresses

Having a mattress I'm happy with has made such a difference to my comfort while sleeping.

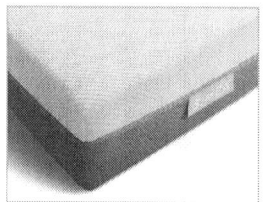

Simba Hybrid Mattress
Simba
https://ibdrelief.com/o/simba

Barefoot shoes

I love these barefoot shoes so much that I now have about 5 pairs and don't wear anything else!

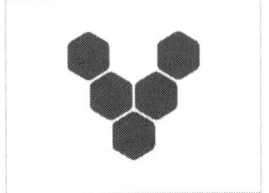

Vivobarefoot
https://ibdrelief.com/o/vivobarefoot

Muscle rollers

I use a foam roller and/or a ball on most days to help with muscle pains. I like products from Trigger Point, but I have also used some from other companies which have been just as good.

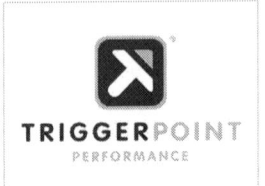

Trigger Point
https://ibdrelief.com/o/trigger-point

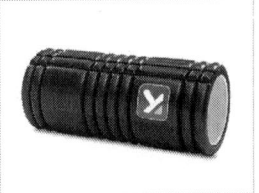

Foam roller
Trigger Point
https://ibdrelief.com/o/roller

Massage Ball
Trigger Point
https://ibdrelief.com/o/massage-ball

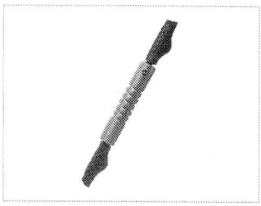

Massage stick
Trigger Point
https://ibdrelief.com/o/massage-stick

Blue light glasses

I pop my blue light glasses on at around 8pm every night to help block out blue light from the various devices around my home. These are the particular glasses that I have:

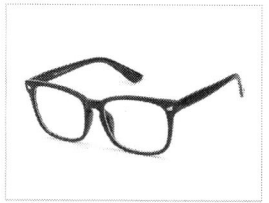

CT82 Horn Oversized Blue Light Blocking Glasses
CGID
https://ibdrelief.com/o/glasses

Eyemask

Great for blocking out light which disturbs my sleep (especially in the summer).

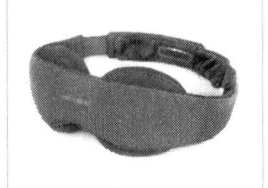

Sleep mask
Manta
https://ibdrelief.com/o/manta

Ear plugs

I have a love-hate relationship with ear plugs. They are great for helping block out noise so I can sleep, but I also find them really annoying and usually take them out around 2am. Ear plugs are such a personal choice and I've tried many on the link below.

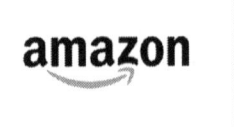

View ear plugs on Amazon
https://ibdrelief.com/o/ear-plugs

Personal care

I use castile soap to make hand soap and shower gel (which I also use to wash my hair) by adding a few drops of essential oils. I also use Green People for products I don't make.

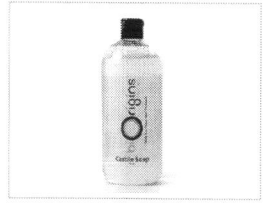

Pure Liquid Castile Soap
Biorigins
https://ibdrelief.com/o/soap

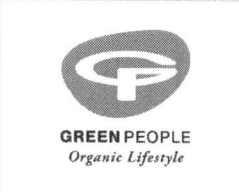

Green People
https://ibdrelief.com/o/green-people

Essential oils

This is the company I buy essential oils from. Their prod-ucts are great, and they are also based near where I live.

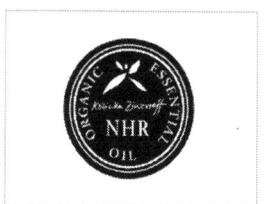

NHR Organic Essential Oils
https://ibdrelief.com/o/nhr

Make up

Ok, so I can't personally recommend this one, but my wife has been using more natural make-up products for a while and loves Green People's range.

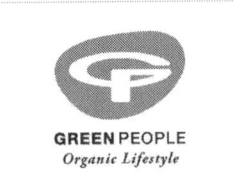

Green People make up
https://ibdrelief.com/o/green-people

Books

Here are some of the books I've found useful or inspiring in my journey.

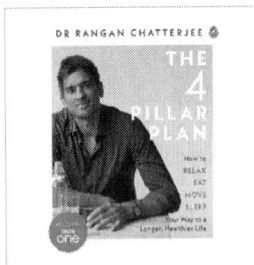

4 Pillar Plan
Rangan Chatterjee
https://ibdrelief.com/o/4-pillar

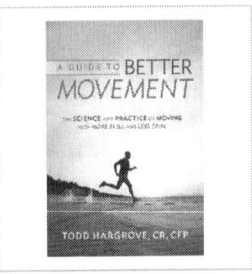

A Guide to Better Movement
Todd Hargrove
https://ibdrelief.com/o/better-movement

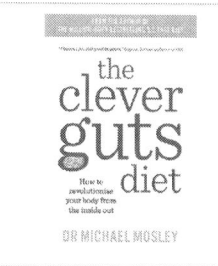

The Clever Guts Diet
Michael Mosley
https://ibdrelief.com/o/clever-guts

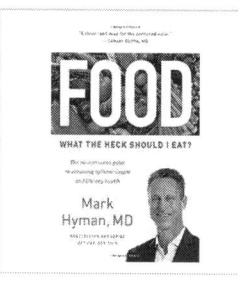

Food: What the Heck Should I Eat
Mark Hyman
https://ibdrelief.com/o/food

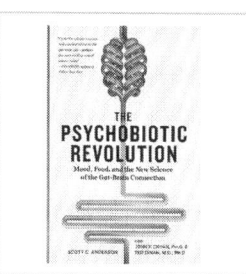

The Psychobiotic Revolution
Scott C Anderson
https://ibdrelief.com/o/psychobiotic

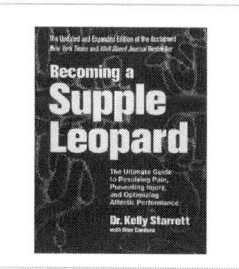

Becoming a Supple Leopard
Kelly Starrett
https://ibdrelief.com/o/leopard

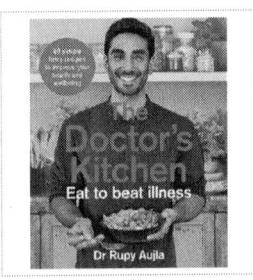

The Doctor's Kitchen - Eat to Beat Illness
Dr Rupy Aujla
https://ibdrelief.com/o/doctors-kitchen

Apps

These are the apps and tech I use.

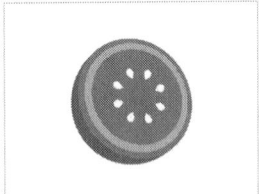

Focus keeper
https://ibdrelief.com/o/focus

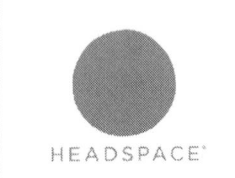

Headspace
https://www.headspace.com

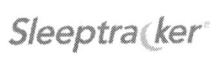

Sleep tracker
https://www.sleeptracker.com

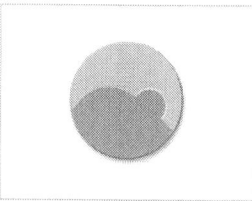

F.lux
https://justgetflux.com

Think Dirty
https://www.thinkdirtyapp.com

Sleepcycle
https://www.sleepcycle.com

About the author

Seb has lived with the long term chronic condition ulcerative colitis since 2008. He has used his experience as a patient and a web agency founder to create ibdrelief.com - a support and information website for people living with inflammatory bowel disease.

He is passionate about improving quality of life for patients living with long term conditions through better information and improved support to self manage their condition. His own disease is currently in remission through using this approach.

Seb is an experienced patient, advocate, entrepreneur, speaker and mentor.

twitter.com/SebTucknott

linkedin.com/in/sebtucknott

instagram.com/sebtucknott

www.sebtucknott.co.uk

Feedback

What did you think of this ebook?

We would love to hear your thoughts about what you've just read.

Email feedback now to info@ibdrelief.com

References

1 Public Health England, https://www.nhs.uk/oneyou/stress#rHPbhhJ8Ym-V19Rj2.97

2 How stress affects your life, American Psychological Association

3 Kiecolt-Glaser, J. & Glaser, R. Stress-induced immune dysfunction: implications for health. Nat Rev Immunol. 2005 Mar;5(3):243-51. doi: 10.1038/nri1571.

4 Thorn, B.E., Pence, L.B., et al. (2007). A randomized clinical trial of targeted cognitive behavioral treatment to reduce catastrophizing in chronic headache sufferers. Journal of Pain 8 , 938-949.

5 Sheldon Cohen, Denise Janicki-Deverts, William J. Doyle, Gregory E. Miller, Ellen Frank, Bruce S. Rabin, and Ronald B. Turner. Chronic stress, glucocorticoid receptor resistance, inflammation, and disease risk. PNAS, April 2, 2012 DOI: 10.1073/pnas.1118355109

6 How stress influences disease: Study reveals inflammation as the culprit, Science Daily, April 2 2012.

7 J E Mawdsley and D S Rampton. Psychological stress in IBD: new insights into pathogenic and therapeutic implications. Gut. 2005 Oct; 54(10): 1481–1491.

8 Bailey MT, Dowd SE, Galley JD, Hufnagle AR, Allen RG, Lyte M. Exposure to a social stressor alters the structure of the intestinal microbiota: implications for stressor-induced immunomodulation. Brain Behav Immun. 2011 Mar;25(3):397-407. doi: 10.1016/j.bbi.2010.10.023. Epub 2010 Oct 30.

9 Public Health England https://www.nhs.uk/oneyou/stress#rHPbhhJ8YmV19Rj2.97

10 Cappuccio FP, D'Elia L, Strazzullo P, Miller MA. Sleep duration and all-cause mortality: a systematic review and meta-analysis of prospective studies. Sleep. 2010 May;33(5):585-92.

11 Kristen L. Knutson. Does inadequate sleep play a role in vulnerability to obesity? American Journal of Human Biology, 2012; 24 (3)

12 Alanna Morris, Dorothy Coverson, Lucy Fike, Yusuf Ahmed, Neli Stoyanova, W. Craig Hooper, Gary Gibbons, Donald Bliwise,Viola Vaccarino, Rebecca Din-Dzietham, and Arshed Quyyumi. Sleep Quality and Duration are Associated with Higher Levels of Inflammatory Biomarkers: the META-Health Study. 23 Mar 2018 Circulation. 2018;122:A17806

13 Z. Ranjbaran, L. Keefer, E. Stepanski, A. Farhadi, A. Keshavarzian. The relevance of sleep abnormalities to chronic inflammatory conditions. Inflammation Research, February 2007, Volume 56, Issue 2, pp 51–57

14 The Science of Sleep. CBS News. https://www.cbsnews.com/news/the-science-of-sleep/

15 Blue light has a dark side. Harvard Health Publishing, Harvard Medical School. https://www.health.harvard.edu/staying-healthy/blue-light-has-a-dark-side

16 Paul D.Loprinzi, Bradley J.Cardina. Association between objectively-measured physical activity and sleep, NHANES 2005–2006. Mental Health and Physical Activity Volume 4, Issue 2, December 2011, Pages 65–69

17 Jounhong Ryan Cho, Eun Yeon Joo, Dae Lim Koo, Seung Bong Hong. Let there be no light: the effect of bedside light on sleep quality and background electroencephalographic rhythms. Sleep Journal December 2013 Volume 14, Issue 12, Pages 1422–1425

18 Kenji Obayashi, Keigo Saeki, Norio Kurumatani. Bedroom Light Exposure at Night and the Incidence of Depressive Symptoms: A Longitudinal Study of the HEIJO-KYO Cohort. American Journal of Epidemiology, Volume 187, Issue 3, 1 March 2018, Pages 427–434

19 Christopher Drake, Ph.D., F.A.A.S.M, Timothy Roehrs, Ph.D., F.A.A.S.M, John Shambroom, B.S, Thomas Roth. Caffeine Effects on Sleep Taken 0, 3, or 6 Hours before Going to Bed. Journal of Clinical Sleep Medicine Volume 09 No. 11

20 Timothy Roehrs, Ph.D, Thomas Roth, Ph.D. Sleep, Sleepiness, and Alcohol Use. National Institute on Alcohol Abuse and Alcoholism.

21 Cappuccio FP, D'Elia L, Strazzullo P, Miller MA. Sleep duration and all-cause mortality: a systematic review and meta-analysis of prospective studies. Sleep. 2010 May;33(5):585-92.

22 Golf SW, Happel O, Graef V, Seim KE. Plasma aldosterone, cortisol and electrolyte concentrations in physical exercise after magnesium supplementation. J Clin Chem Clin Biochem. 1984 Nov;22(11):717-21

23 Didier Chollet, Paul Franken, Yvette Raffin, Alain Malafosse, Jean Widmer and Mehdi Tafti. Blood and brain magnesium in inbred mice and their correlation with sleep quality. American Journal of Physiology Volume 279 Issue 6 December 2000 Pages R2173-R2178

24 John H.Lee MD, James H.O'Keefe MD, David Bell MD, Donald D.Hensrud MD, MPH, Michael F.Holick MD, PhD. Vitamin D Deficiency: An Important, Common, and Easily Treatable Cardiovascular Risk Factor? Journal of the American College of Cardiology Volume 52, Issue 24, 9 December 2008, Pages 1949-1956

25 Gominak SC, Stumpf WE. The world epidemic of sleep disorders is linked to vitamin D deficiency. Med Hypotheses. 2012 Aug;79(2):132-5. doi: 10.1016/j.mehy.2012.03.031. Epub 2012 May 13

26 Emanuela Esposito and Salvatore Cuzzocrea. Antiinflammatory Activity of Melatonin in Central Nervous System. Curr Neuropharmacol. 2010 Sep; 8(3): 228-242

27 Tharwat S Kandil, Amany A Mousa, Ahmed A El-Gendy, and Amr M Abbas. The potential therapeutic effect of melatonin in gastro-esophageal reflux disease. BMC Gastroenterol. 2010; 10: 7. Published online 2010 Jan 18

28 Palmer C, Bik EM, DiGiulio DB, Relman DA, Brown PO. Development of the human infant intestinal microbiota. PLoS Biol. 2007;5:e177. [PMC free article] [PubMed]

29 Jun Sun , Eugene B. Chang. Exploring gut microbes in human health and disease: Pushing the envelope. Genes & Diseases. Volume 1, Issue 2, December 2014, Pages 132-139

30 Z. Ranjbaran, L. Keefer, E. Stepanski, A. Farhadi, A. Keshavarzian. The relevance of sleep abnormalities to chronic inflammatory conditions. Inflammation Research, February 2007, Volume 56, Issue 2, pp 51-57

31 Guy Sisson, Bu Hayee, Ingvar Bjarnason. Assessment of a Multi Strain Probiotic (Symprove) in IBD. Gastroenterology April 2015 Volume 148, Issue 4, Supplement 1, Page S-531

32 Andrew C. Dukowicz MD, Brian E. Lacy PhD, MD, and Gary M. Levine, MD. Small Intestinal Bacterial Overgrowth: A Comprehensive Review. Gastroenterol Hepatol (N Y). 2007 Feb; 3(2): 112–122

33 Rana SV, Sharma S, Malik A, Kaur J, Prasad KK, Sinha SK, Singh K. Small intestinal bacterial overgrowth and orocecal transit time in patients of inflammatory bowel disease. Dig Dis Sci. 2013 Sep;58(9):2594-8. doi: 10.1007/s10620-013-2694-x. Epub 2013 May 7

34 Jochen Klaus, Ulrike Spaniol, Guido Adler, Richard A Mason, Max Reinshagen and Christian von Tirpitz C. Small intestinal bacterial overgrowth mimicking acute flare as a pitfall in patients with Crohn's Disease. BMC Gastroenterology 2009 9:61

35 Sandro Drago et al. Gliadin, zonulin and gut permeability: Effects on celiac and non-celiac intestinal mucosa and intestinal cell lines. Scandinavian Journal of Gastroenterology Volume 41, 2006 - Issue 4

36 Alessio Fasano. Intestinal Permeability and Its Regulation by Zonulin: Diagnostic and Therapeutic Implications. Clinical Gastroenterology and Hepatology Volume 10, Issue 10, October 2012, Pages 1096-1100

37 Herfarth HH, Martin CF, Sandler RS, Kappelman MD, Long MD. Prevalence of a gluten-free diet and improvement of clinical symptoms in patients with inflammatory bowel diseases. Inflamm Bowel Dis. 2014 Jul;20(7):1194-7

38 Article in Medical News Today - http://www.medicalnewstoday.com/articles/313514.php

39 Everything you need to know about lactose intolerance. New Scientist. 23 July 2015.

40 C. Menezes, R. Rocha, F. Coqueiro, M. Lopes, P. Nunes, L. Sales, C. Factum, N. Almeida, G. Santana, B. César da Silva. Lactose intolerance in inflammatory bowel disease patients. Poster presentation, ECCO 2013.

41 Sophia J. Oak & Rajesh Jha. The effects of probiotics in lactose intolerance: A systematic review. Critical Reviews in Food Science and Nutrition. 9 Feb 2018

42 Eric Robinson, Paul Aveyard, Amanda Daley, Kate Jolly, Amanda Lewis, Deborah Lycett, Suzanne Higgs. Eating attentively: a systematic review and meta-analysis of

the effect of food intake memory and awareness on eating. The American Journal of Clinical Nutrition, Volume 97, Issue 4, 1 April 2013, Pages 728–742

43 The Nobel Prize in Physiology or Medicine 2016. Press release

44 Mark D. DeBoer. Use of Ghrelin as a Treatment for Inflammatory Bowel Disease: Mechanistic Considerations. International Journal of Peptides. Published online 2011 Aug 9.

45 Eveline Deloose, Pieter Janssen, Inge Depoortere, Jan Tack. Nature Reviews Gastro-enterology & Hepatology. Volume 9, pages 271–285 (2012)

46 Aeberli I, Gerber PA, Hochuli M, Kohler S, Haile SR, Gouni-Berthold I, Berthold HK, Spinas GA, Berneis K. Low to moderate sugar-sweetened beverage consumption impairs glucose and lipid metabolism and promotes inflammation in healthy young men: a randomized controlled trial. Am J Clin Nutr. 2011 Aug;94(2):479-85. doi: 10.3945/ajcn.111.013540. Epub 2011 Jun 15.

47 Faizan Jameel, Melinda Phang, Lisa G Wood, Manohar L Garg. Acute effects of feeding fructose, glucose and sucrose on blood lipid levels and systemic inflammation. Lipids Health Dis. 2014; 13: 195.

48 Suez J et al. Artificial sweeteners induce glucose intolerance by altering the gut microbiota. Nature. 2014 Oct 9;514(7521):181-6. doi: 10.1038/nature13793. Epub 2014 Sep 17

49 Dorin Harpaz, Loo Pin Yeo, Francesca Cecchini, Trish H. P. Koon, Ariel Kushmaro, Alfred I. Y. Tok, Robert S. Marks, Evgeni Eltzov. Measuring Artificial Sweeteners Tox-icity Using a Bioluminescent Bacterial Panel. Molecules 2018, 23(10), 2454

50 Marco Ardesia, Guido Ferlazzo, Walter Fries. Vitamin D and Inflammatory Bowel Disease. Biomed Res Int. 2015; 2015: 470805

51 Toufic A Kabbani, Ioannis E Koutroubakis, Robert E Schoen, Claudia Ramos-Rivers, Nilesh Shah, Jason Swoger, Miguel Regueiro, Arthur Barrie, Marc Schwartz, Jana G Hashash, Leonard Baidoo, Michael A Dunn and David G Binion. Association of Vitamin D Level With Clinical Status in Inflammatory Bowel Disease: A 5-Year Longitudinal Study. The American Journal of Gastroenterology 111, 712-719 (May 2016)

52 Public Health England. Press release, 21 July 2016.

53 Schwalfenberg GK, Genuis SJ.The Importance of Magnesium in Clinical Healthcare. Scientifica (Cairo). 2017;2017:4179326. doi: 10.1155/2017/4179326. Epub 2017 Sep 28.

54 Galland L. Magnesium and inflammatory bowel disease. Magnesium. 1988;7(2):78-83

55 Pietro Dulbecco and Vincenzo Savarino. Therapeutic potential of curcumin in digestive diseases. World J Gastroenterol. 2013 Dec 28; 19(48): 9256-9270.

56 John H.Lee MD, James H.O'Keefe MD, David Bell MD, Donald D.Hensrud MD, MPH, Michael F.Holick MD, PhD. Vitamin D Deficiency: An Important, Common, and Easily Treatable Cardiovascular Risk Factor? Journal of the American College of Cardiology Volume 52, Issue 24, 9 December 2008, Pages 1949-1956

57 RadhaKrishna Rao and Geetha Samak. Role of Glutamine in Protection of Intestinal Epithelial Tight Junctions. J Epithel Biol Pharmacol. 2012 Jan; 5(Suppl 1-M7): 47-54.

58 RadhaKrishna Rao and Geetha Samak. Role of Glutamine in Protection of Intestinal Epithelial Tight Junctions. J Epithel Biol Pharmacol. 2012 Jan; 5(Suppl 1-M7): 47-54.

59 Published Studies on the Efficacy of MSM (methylsulfonylmethane).

60 Barmaki S, Bohlooli S, Khoshkhahesh F, Nakhostin-Roohi B. Effect of methylsulfonylmethane supplementation on exercise - Induced muscle damage and total antioxidant capacity. J Sports Med Phys Fitness. 2012 Apr;52(2):170-4.

61 Kalman DS, Feldman S, Scheinberg AR, Krieger DR, Bloomer RJ. Influence of methylsulfonylmethane on markers of exercise recovery and performance in healthy men: a pilot study. J Int Soc Sports Nutr. 2012 Sep 27;9(1):46. doi: 10.1186/1550-2783-9-46.

62 Z. Khan, C. Macdonald, A. C. Wicks, M. P. Holt, D. Floyd, S. Ghosh, N. A. Wright, R. J. Playford. Use of the 'nutriceutical', bovine colostrum, for the treatment of distal colitis: results from an initial study. Alimentary Pharmacology and Therapeutics, Volume 16, Issue 11, November 2002, Pages 1917-1922

63 Caldarini de Bustos MI, Schiffrin EJ, Ogawa de Furuya K, Caccamo DV, Ledesma

de Paolo MI, Celener D, Bustos-Fernández L. Prevention of carrageenan-induced ulcerative colitis in the guinea pig by serum of bovine colostrum. Medicina (B Aires). 1987;47(3):273-7.

64 Z. Khan, C. Macdonald, A. C. Wicks, M. P. Holt, D. Floyd, S. Ghosh, N. A. Wright, R. J. Playford. Use of the 'nutriceutical', bovine colostrum, for the treatment of distal colitis: results from an initial study. Alimentary Pharmacology and Therapeutics, Volume 16, Issue 11, November 2002, Pages 1917-1922

65 Aleksandra Pituch-Zdanowska, Aleksandra Banaszkiewicz, and Piotr Albrecht. The role of dietary fibre in inflammatory bowel disease. Prz Gastroenterol. 2015; 10(3): 135-141.

66 Carol S. Brotherton, Christopher A. Martin, Millie D. Long, Michael D. Kappelman, Robert S. Sandler. Avoidance of Fiber Is Associated With Greater Risk of Crohn's Disease Flare in a 6-Month Period. Clinical Gastroenterology and Hepatology, August 2016 Volume 14, Issue 8, Pages 1130-1136

67 Celestine Wong, Philip J. Harris, Lynnette R. Ferguson. Potential Benefits of Dietary Fibre Intervention in Inflammatory Bowel Disease. Int. J. Mol. Sci. 2016, 17(6), 919; doi:10.3390/ijms17060919

68 Gonçalves P, Martel F. Butyrate and colorectal cancer: the role of butyrate transport. Curr Drug Metab. 2013 Nov;14(9):994-1008.

69 Kelly Cushing, David M Alvarado & Matthew A Ciorba. Butyrate and Mucosal Inflammation: New Scientific Evidence Supports Clinical Observation. Clinical and Translational Gastroenterology volume 6, page e108 (2015)

70 Jan Bilski, Bartosz Brzozowski, Agnieszka Mazur-Bialy, Zbigniew Sliwowski, and Tomasz Brzozowski. The Role of Physical Exercise in Inflammatory Bowel Disease. BioMed Research International. Volume 2014 (2014), Article ID 429031, 14 pages

71 Peters HP, De Vries WR, Vanberge-Henegouwen GP, Akkermans LM. Potential benefits and hazards of physical activity and exercise on the gastrointestinal tract. Gut. 2001 Mar;48(3):435-9. PMID: 11171839

72 Eun Ran Kim and Dong Kyung Chang. Colorectal cancer in inflammatory bowel disease: The risk, pathogenesis, prevention and diagnosis. World J Gastroenterol. 2014

Aug 7; 20(29): 9872–9881.

73 Stoyan Dimitrov, Elaine Hulteng, Suzi Hong. Inflammation and exercise: Inhibition of monocytic intracellular TNF production by acute exercise via β2-adrenergic activation. Brain, Behavior, and Immunity, volume 61, March 2017, pages 60–68

74 Ho GW. Lower gastrointestinal distress in endurance athletes. Curr Sports Med Rep. 2009 Mar-Apr;8(2):85-91.

75 Jonathan P. Little, Mary E. Jung, Amy E. Wright, Wendi Wright, Ralph J.F. Manders. Effects of high-intensity interval exercise versus continuous moderate-intensity exercise on postprandial glycemic control assessed by continuous glucose monitoring in obese adults. Applied Physiology, Nutrition, and Metabolism, 2014, 39(7): 835–841

76 Ramos JS, Dalleck LC, Tjonna AE, Beetham KS, Coombes JS. The impact of high-intensity interval training versus moderate-intensity continuous training on vascular function: a systematic review and meta-analysis. Sports Med. 2015 May;45(5):679-92. doi: 10.1007/s40279-015-0321-z.

77 Robinson MM, Dasari S, Konopka AR, Johnson ML, Manjunatha S, Esponda RR, Carter RE, Lanza IR, Nair KS. Enhanced Protein Translation Underlies Improved Metabolic and Physical Adaptations to Different Exercise Training Modes in Young and Old Humans. Cell Metab. 2017 Mar 7;25(3):581-592. doi: 10.1016/j.cmet.2017.02.009.

78 M. A. Nimmo, M. Leggate, J. L. Viana, J. A. King. The effect of physical activity on mediators of inflammation. Diabetes, Obesity and Metabolism. Volume 15, issue s3, September 2013, pages 51-60

79 Allen JM, Mailing LJ, Niemiro GM, Moore R, Cook MD, White BA, Holscher HD, Woods JA. Exercise Alters Gut Microbiota Composition and Function in Lean and Obese Humans. Med Sci Sports Exerc. 2018 Apr;50(4):747-757. doi: 10.1249/MSS.0000000000001495.

80 Evangelia Legaki and Maria Gazouli. Influence of environmental factors in the development of inflammatory bowel diseases. World J Gastrointest Pharmacol Ther. 2016 Feb 6; 7(1): 112–125.

81 PREdiCCT study

82 Kyriaki Remoundou and Phoebe Koundouri. Environmental Effects on Public Health: An Economic Perspective. Int J Environ Res Public Health. 2009 Aug; 6(8): 2160–2178.

83 World Health Organisation: Chlorine in Drinking Water

84 World Health Organisation: Ambient (outdoor) air quality and health

85 Annual report of the Chief Medical Officer 2017: Health Impacts of All Pollution – what do we know?

86 United States Environmental Protection Agency: Volatile Organic Compounds' Impact on Indoor Air Quality

87 World Health Organisation, Europe: Dampness and Mould

88 World Health Organisation, Europe: Dampness and Mould - Health risks, prevention and remedial actions

89 World Health Organisation: Endocrine disrupting Chemicals

90 Kevin M. Rice, Ernest M. Walker, Jr, Miaozong Wu, Chris Gillette, and Eric R. Blough. Environmental Mercury and Its Toxic Effects. J Prev Med Public Health. 2014 Mar; 47(2): 74–83.

91 World Health Organisation: International Programme on Chemical Safety - Mercury

48173081R00105

Printed in Poland
by Amazon Fulfillment
Poland Sp. z o.o., Wrocław